浙江省普通高校"十三五"新形态教材
高等医学院国际化英语教学教材
职业教育数字化融媒体特色教材

（英文版）

NURSING SIMULATIONS FOR COMPREHENSIVE TRAINING

涉外护理情景模拟综合实训

袁浩斌　王　薇　费素定◎主　审
刘桂娟　葛　炜◎主　编
吴珊珊　陈　燕　郭玲玲◎副主编

ZHEJIANG UNIVERSITY PRESS
浙江大学出版社
国家一级出版社
全国百佳图书出版单位

编委会

主　审　袁浩斌　王　薇　费素定

主　编　刘桂娟　葛　炜

副主编　吴珊珊　陈　燕　郭玲玲

编　委　（按姓氏拼音排序）

陈鸿尔　（宁波市医疗中心李惠利医院）

陈巍阳　（深圳卓正医疗投资咨询有限公司）

陈　燕　（宁波卫生职业技术学院）

葛　炜　（宁波卫生职业技术学院）

郭玲玲　（江苏医药职业学院）

林　凯　（浙江省医疗服务管理评价中心）

刘桂娟　（宁波卫生职业技术学院）

梅一宁　（宁波卫生职业技术学院）

乔　乔　（宁波卫生职业技术学院）

王锡唯　（中国科学院大学宁波华美医院）

邬维娜　（杭州医学院）

吴珊珊　（宁波卫生职业技术学院）

徐　倩　（宁波大学医学院附属医院）

前 言

随着社会的变迁，护理专业的发展迎来了巨大的挑战。全球化进程的加快使得护理人员面对的服务群体更加多元，而英语作为全球范围内通用的交流工具，在促进不同文化背景的医护患交流中日益显现出重要作用。

本教材以英文语境为基础，以职业能力培养为主线，按场景、任务搭建教材框架，以临床案例为载体，基于实际工作过程设计学习任务。教材以整合场景、案例导入、完成典型工作任务的形式，将院前急救、成人护理、母婴护理及基础护理等内容有机组合，呈现临床各科最常用、最基本的知识和技能，旨在提升学生实训技能，同时提高其英语的临床实际应用能力。

本教材在内容的选择和安排上坚持以学生为主体，教材设计体现涉外护理工作岗位需求，强化临床涉外护理工作中常涉及的词汇和语句。教材图文并茂，有背景知识介绍、操作流程展示，以实拍图片和简洁对话框的形式突出要点，并结合国际护士执业水平考试（ISPN）课程内容，为学生提供适应涉外护理工作岗位的学习资源。

本教材由涉外护理专业专、兼职教师团队及浙江省内外兄弟院校教师共同编写，是宁波卫生职业技术学院首批"岗位胜任力系列教材"之一，可供护理专业、涉外护理专业选用。

本教材的编写得到了澳门理工学院袁浩斌博士、浙江大学附属第一医院王薇博士和宁波卫生职业技术学院护理学院院长费素定教授的倾力指导，在此深表谢意！

编者首次尝试全英文编写，水平有限，教材中难免存在不妥之处，恳请广大师生批评指正。

编 者

2022 年 3 月

Comprehensive Case:
A Car Accident

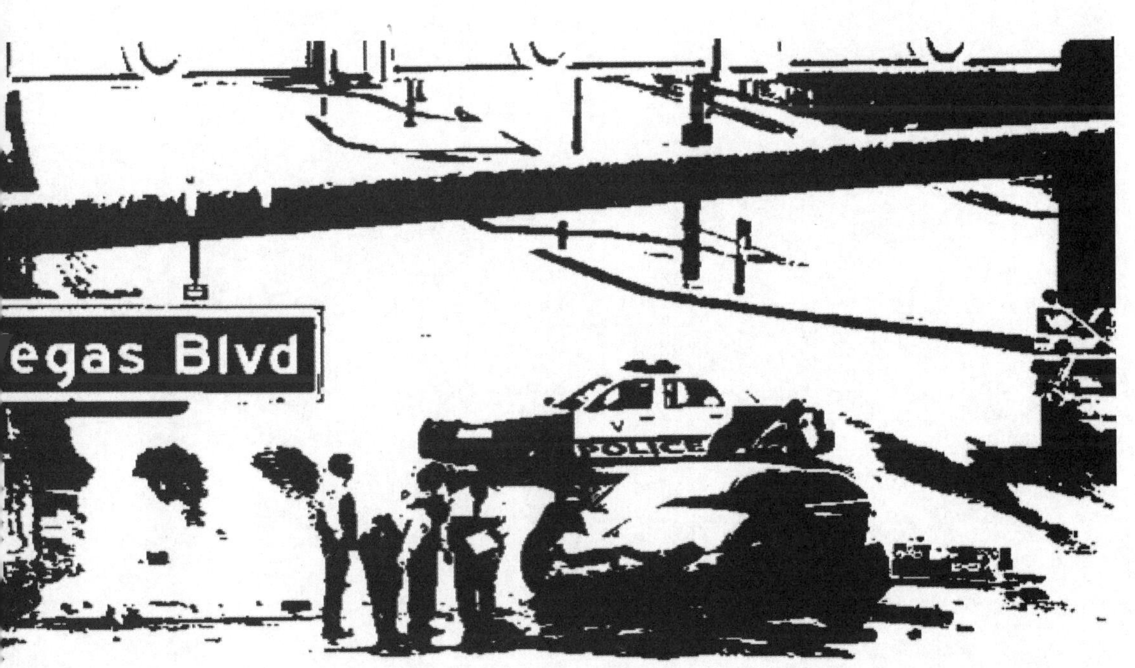

A severe car accident occurred at 12:00 BST on Sunday between Las Vegas Blvd and Kingsford Railway Bridge. A female drove a sedan traveling north at a high speed. It ran through a red light and crashed with a Toyota SUV traveling west. A pedestrian and the SUV driver were seriously injured. All the drivers and passengers on the cars were taken to the nearest hospital for further treatment. Police appealed for anyone who saw the crash or the cars traveling in either direction beforehand to come forward.

• Client 1

Mary is a 28-year-old female driver in this severe car crash. The surveillance showed this accident was directly caused by her dangerous driving behavior. She was found without any obvious injury, although her forehead hit the steering wheel in the accident.

• Client 2

David is a 45-year-old male pedestrian involved in this accident. Mary's car hit him laterally when he was walking across the road. He was unconscious immediately.

• Client 3

Anne is the 56-year-old driver of the SUV, who alongside her husband Jack were taking their 24-week-pregnant daughter Catherine to the hospital for a prenatal physical examination. Anne's right calf was stuck in the car and her right arm was bleeding profusely. She also complained of severe pain in the left abdomen.

• Client 4

Jack is a 65-year-old man with a 40 years' history of smoking and has been diagnosed with COPD for 5 years. He was in the back seat and had no injury.

• Client 5

Catherine is a 32-year-old pregnant lady. She was heading to the hospital for her 24 weeks gestational examination. She was in the back seat and thus avoided injury from the broken glass.

• Client 6

Lucy is Catherine's 3-month-old niece. She was sitting in the safety seat in the back seat with her aunt. She kept crying after the crash though injuries were found. Catherine decided to bring Lucy to the hospital for a comprehensive check-up.

（吴珊珊）

Scenario One
First Aid

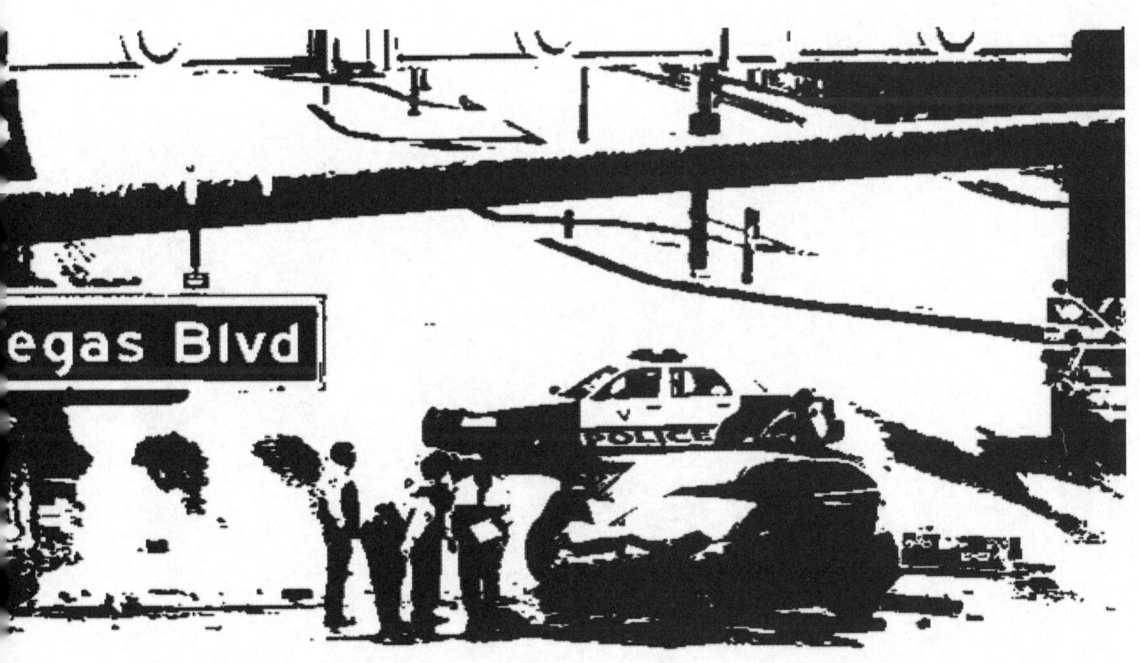

TASK 1

Cardiopulmonary Resuscitation

Learning Outcomes

This task will provide students with opportunities to:

- Clarify risk factors related to heart arrest.
- Perform cardiopulmonary resuscitation correctly and instantly.
- Cooperate and communicate with other health professionals effectively.
- Complete relative nursing documents appropriately.

Scenario

David is a 45-year-old male pedestrian involved in this accident. Mary's car hit him laterally when he was walking across the road. He immediately lost his consciousness, pulse, and breath.

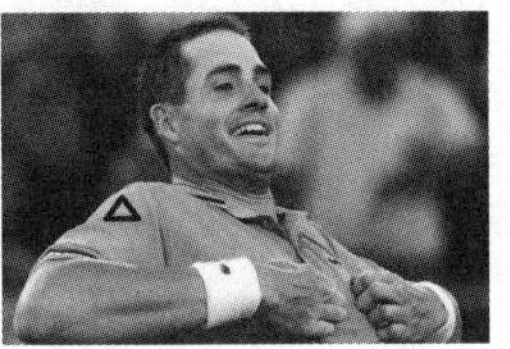

1-1 CPR PPT

Background

Cardiopulmonary resuscitation (CPR) is an emergency procedure performed in an effort to manually preserve intact brain function until further measures are taken to restore spontaneous blood circulation and breath of someone who is in cardiac arrest.

Sudden cardiac arrest may be caused by coronary heart disease, other cardiac or non-cardiac conditions which may include trauma, bleeding (such as gastrointestinal bleeding, aortic rupture, or intracranial hemorrhage), overdose, drowning and pulmonary embolism. Cardiac arrest can also be caused by poisoning. The risk factors include smoking, lack of physical exercise, obesity and diabetes, as well as family history.

CPR is indicated in unresponsive persons with no breathing or abnormal breathing, for example, agonal respiration. According to the American Heart Association (AHA) and International Liaison Committee on Resuscitation Guidelines, CPR involves chest compression for 5—6 cm deep and at a rate of 100—120 times per minute to create artificial circulation by manually pumping blood from the heart to the body. The rescuer may also provide breaths by either exhaling into the patient's mouth or nose or using a device that pushes air into the patient's lung. This process of externally providing ventilation is termed artificial respiration. Current recommendations emphasize high-quality chest compression over artificial respiration; a simplified CPR method involving chest compression only is recommended for untrained rescuers.

CPR alone is unlikely to restart the heart. Its main purpose is to restore the partial flow of oxygenated blood to the brain and the heart. The objective is to delay tissue death and extend the brief window of opportunity for a successful resuscitation without permanent brain damage. Administration of an electric shock to the patient's heart, termed defibrillation, is usually needed to restore a viable heart rhythm. Defibrillation is effective only for certain heart rhythms, namely ventricular fibrillation or pulseless ventricular tachycardia, rather than asystole or pulseless electrical activity. In general, CPR is continued until the patient's return of spontaneous circulation (ROSC) or dead is declared.

1-2 CPR 讲解视频

Process

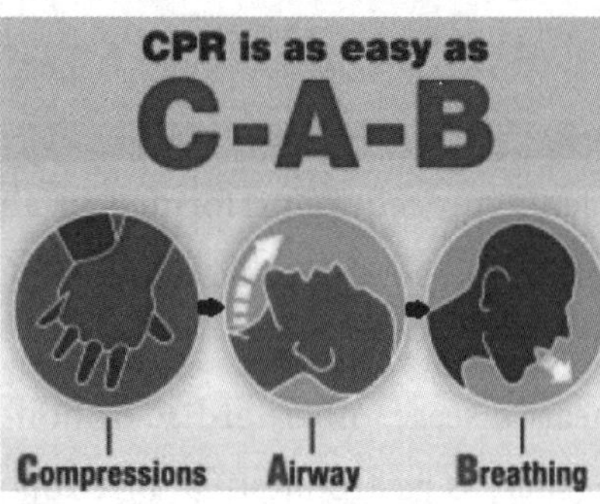

[Compressions]

Push hard and fast on the center of the victim's chest.

[Airway]

Tilt the victim's head back and lift the chin to open the airway.

[Breathing]

Give mouth-to-mouth resuscitation or use a device to rescue breath.

Procedure

1-3 CPR 操作视频

Step 1: Assess environment and prepare yourself.

- The environment is safe. The rescuers apply gloves and face shields, if available.

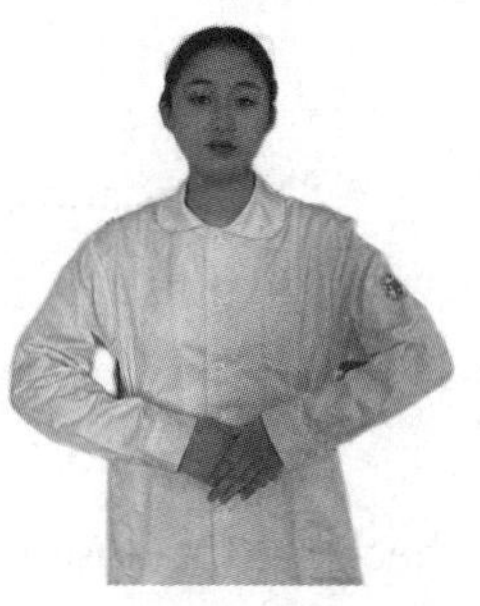

"The environment is safe. Self-protections are ready."

Step 2: Assess awareness.

□ Gently shake the victim's shoulders and ask "Are you OK?" Be alert to the potential head or neck injury.

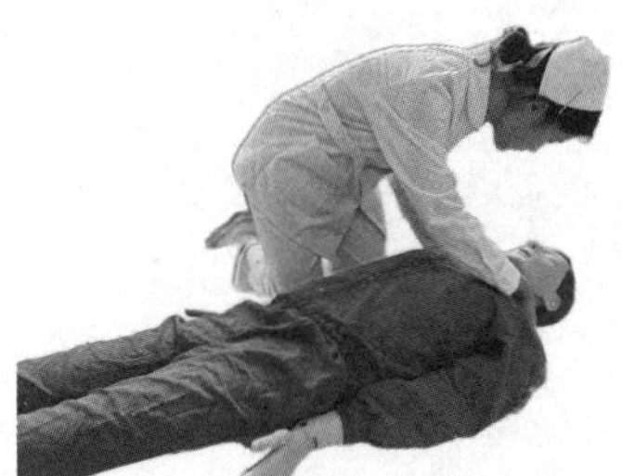

"Hey! Hey! Are you OK? No consciousness."

□ For the Health Care Practitioner (HCP), determining the victim's unresponsiveness is the first.

Step 3: Initiate EMSS.

□ EMSS is the abbreviation of emergency medical service system. Call 120 the moment you realize the victim can not be waked up and doesn't seem to be breathing right.

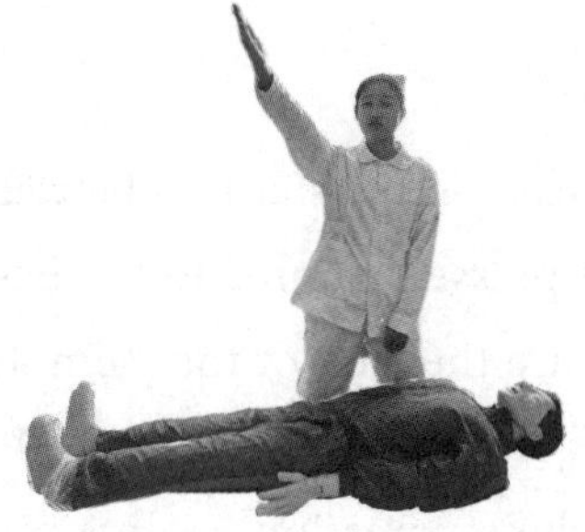

"Help! Help! He/She needs first aid.
Please call 120 and give me feedback.
Please go to fetch AED."

Step 4: Determine breath and pulse.

□ Set eyes on the thorax and the abdomen to observe whether there are ups and downs. CPR guidelines recommend that laying persons should not be instructed to check the pulse, while giving healthcare professionals the option to check a pulse. To correctly determine, please assess for 5 to 10 seconds.

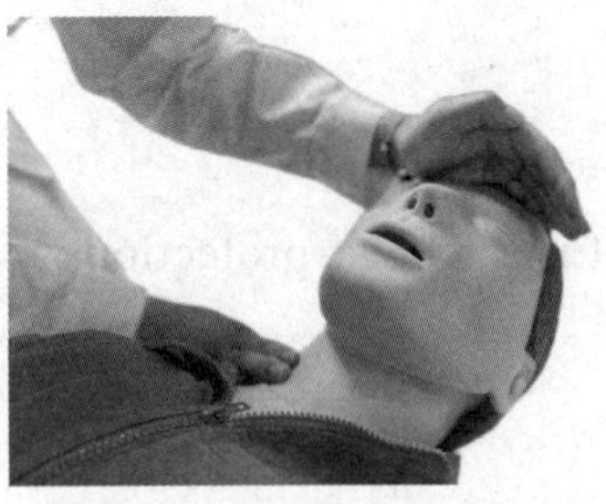

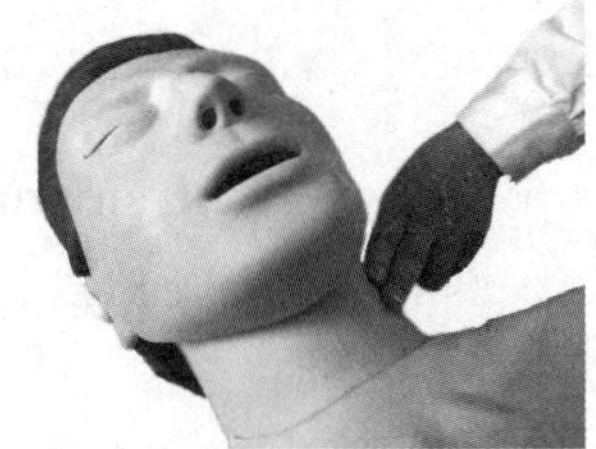

"No ups and downs!
No pulse!"

▫ Palpate the carotid artery to assess circulation, and always check for the absence of pulse before beginning chest compression.

Step 5: Place the victim in a supine position.

▫ Place the victim in a supine position on a firm and flat surface (logroll the victim, using spine precautions), untie the collor, and loosen the belt.

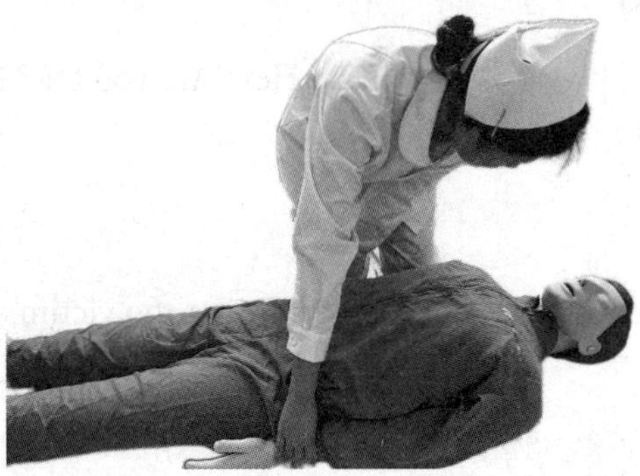

Step 6: Perform chest compression.

▫ Chest compression landmark: center of the chest, between the nipples; middle and lower 1/2 of sternum.

▫ Chest compression method:

(1) The rescuer uses two hands: The base of one palm is placed on the sternum between the two nipples, and the other hand is overlapped and pressed parallel to the back of the hand. The rescuer should straighten the elbows, use the base of the palm, lift the fingers away from the chest wall, press for 5—6cm, and the frequency is 100—120 times/min. Allow the chest to fully recoil after each compression, maintaining cortinuous regular compressions.

(2) The rescuer should push hard and fast and avoid interruption until the AED is in place and ready to analyze the heart rate. When it is time to give artificial respiration, do it quickly and get right back on the chest.

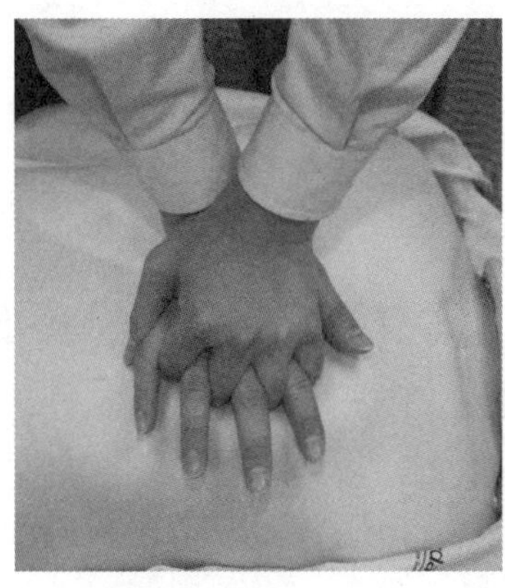

"One, two, three, four... thirty!"

Step 7: Open the airway.

- Wipe out any obvious foreign matter.
- Open the airway using the head tilt-chin lift or the jaw thrust maneuver.

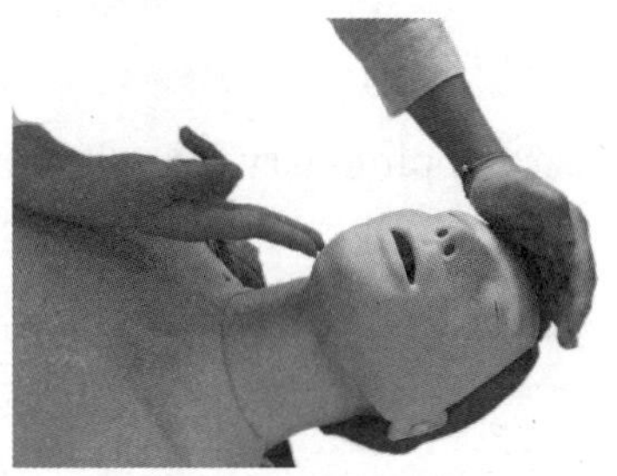

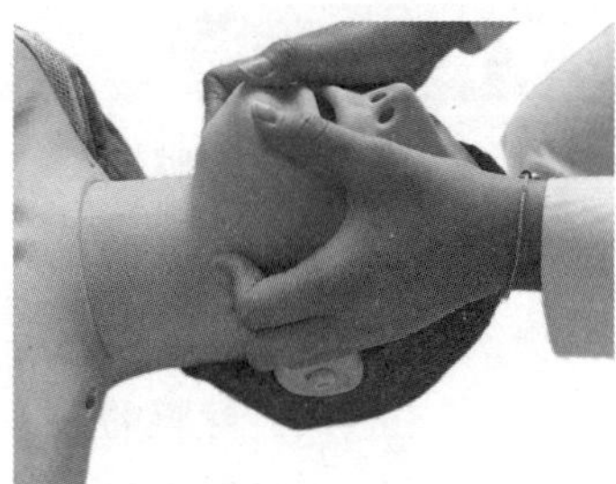

Step 8: Initiate breathing.

- Keep the airway open.
- Deliver two initial effective breaths (breaths that cause a visible chest rise) to the victim, mouth to mouth with noses closed at a rate of 10 to 12 breaths per minute.
- The compression-to-ventilation ratio is 30 : 2 (for either one or two rescuers).
- Pinch the victim's nostrils as you blow and relax as you exhale. Every time you blow, you should tightly wrap the victim's mouth, pinch the nose, and take more than 1 second to give a tidal volume of 500—600 ml that is enough to lift the chest.

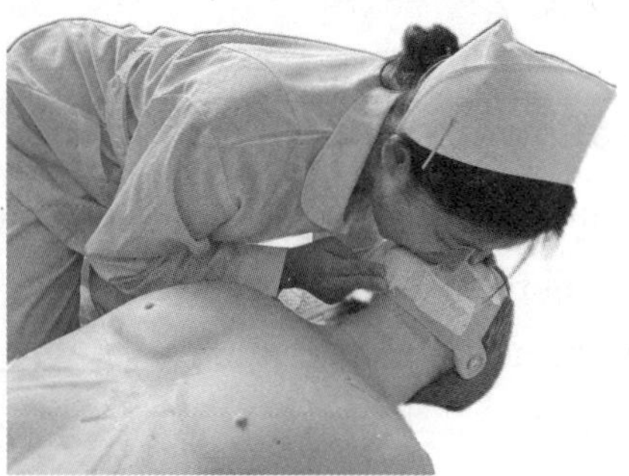

Step 9: Reassess the victim.

- After five circles of 30∶2, reassess the victim's consciousness, breathing, and pulse. If there is none, continue compressing and breathing again.

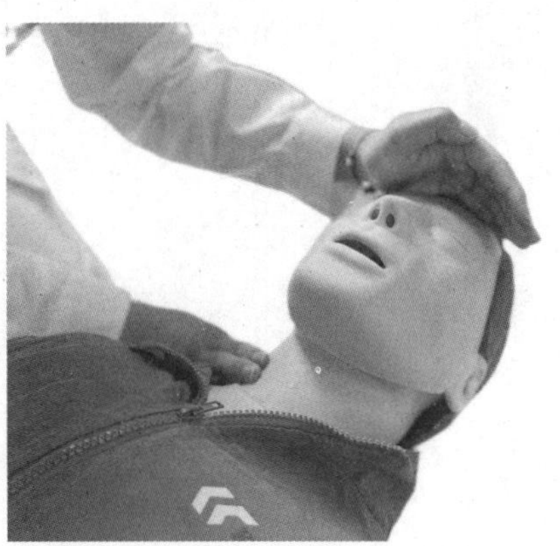

Words and Phrases

cardi(o)-	心、心脏的	cardiopulmonary resuscitation (CPR)	心肺复苏术
atri(o)-	心、心脏的	head tilt-chin lift	仰头举颏法（压额提颏法）
ventricul(o)-	血管的	jaw thrust maneuver	抬下颌法
valv(o)-, valvul(o)-	瓣膜的	chest compression	胸外心脏按压
cardiac arrest	心搏骤停	artificial circulation	人工循环
agonal respiration	叹息样呼吸	artificial respiration	人工呼吸
automated external defibrillator (AED)	自动体外除颤仪	defibrillation	除颤
basic life support (BLS)	基础生命支持	ventricular fibrillation	心室颤动
advanced cardiovascular life support (ACLS)	高级生命支持		

Learning Activities

Part I Choose the best answer for each question.

1. A nurse on the day shift walks into a patient's room and finds the patient unresponsive. The patient has no breath and pulse, and the nurse immediately calls out for help. Which of the following is the next nursing action? ________

A. Open the airway.

B. Give the client oxygen.

C. Start chest compression.

D. Ventilate with a mouth-to-mask device.

2. A nurse witnesses a neighbor's husband sustain a fall from the roof of his house. The nurse rushes to the victim and determines the need to open the airway. Which method does the nurse use for openning the airway of this victim? ________

A. Flexed position.

B. Head tilt-chin lift.

C. Jaw thrust maneuver.

D. Modified head tilt-chin lift.

3. Which of the following is a correct guideline for adult CPR for a health care provider? ________

A. One breath should be given for every 5 compressions.

B. Two breaths should be given for every 15 compressions.

C. Initially, two quick breaths should be given as rapidly as possible.

D. Each rescue breath should be given over 1 second and should produce a visible chest rise.

4. A nurse is performing CPR on an adult client. When performing chest compression, the nurse should depress the sternum for ________.

A. 0.75 to 1 inch

B. 0.5 to 0.75 inch

C. 1.5 to 2 inches

D. 2.5 to 3 inches

5. A nurse is performing CPR on a man. When performing chest compression, the nurse compresses for ________.

A. 60 to 80 times per minute

B. 80 to 100 times per minute

C. 100 to 120 times per minute

D. 120 to 140 times per minute

6. A nurse is performing CPR on a 7-year-old child. How many breaths per minute does the nurse deliver to the child? ________.

A. 6

B. 8

C. 10

D. 20

7. A nurse is performing CPR on a man. How many breaths per minute does the nurse deliver to the man?________.

A. 6

B. 8

C. 10

D. 20

8. A nurse is performing CPR on an infant. When performing chest compression, the nurse compresses for________.

A. 60 to 80 times per minute

B. 80 to 100 times per minute

C. 100 to 120 times per minute

D. 120 to 140 times per minute

9. A nurse is teaching CPR to nursing students. The nurse asks a student to describe the reason why blind finger sweeps are avoided in infants. If the student makes the statement that ________ the nurse determines that the student understands this reason.

A. "The object may have been swallowed,"

B. "The infant may bite down on the finger,"

C. "The mouth is too small to see the object,"

D. "The object may be forced back farther into the throat,"

10. A nursing student is asked to describe the correct steps for performing abdominal thrusts on an unconscious adult. Number in order of priority the steps for performing this procedure. (Number 1 is the first step and number 5 is the last step.)

________ Open the airway.

________ Attempt ventilation.

________ Assess unconsciousness.

________ Perform abdominal thrusts.

________ Look in the mouth and remove the object blocking the airway if seen.

Part II Case study.

Case Scenario

In less than 30 seconds Heidi Kuite's 10-month-old son silently slipped under 6 inches of bath water. Zayden had gotten out of his safety bath seat when Heidi went to get a towel. Seconds later, he was submerged. Heidi's husband Anthony returned to check on the baby and quickly pulled him out of the water. Zayden's lips were blue and he wasn't breathing. Anthony started giving breaths and called his wife for help. Heidi had taken a CPR course four years earlier and knew what to do: immediately start CPR. Meanwhile, a family friend called 911.

Task: Clarify the differences between adult CPR and infant CPR.

（刘桂娟　徐　倩）

TASK 2

Trauma Management

Learning Outcomes

This task will provide students with opportunities to:

- Clarify risk factors related to trauma.
- Understand principles of first aid in trauma care.
- Perform trauma management correctly and smoothly in emergent situation.
- Cooperate and communicate with other health professionals effectively and efficiently.
- Complete relative nursing documents appropriately.

Scenario

Anne is a 56-year-old driver of an SUV. She was taking her 24-week-pregnant daughter Catherine to the hospital for a prenatal physical examination. When the car accident happened, her right calf was stuck in the car and her right arm was bleeding profusely.

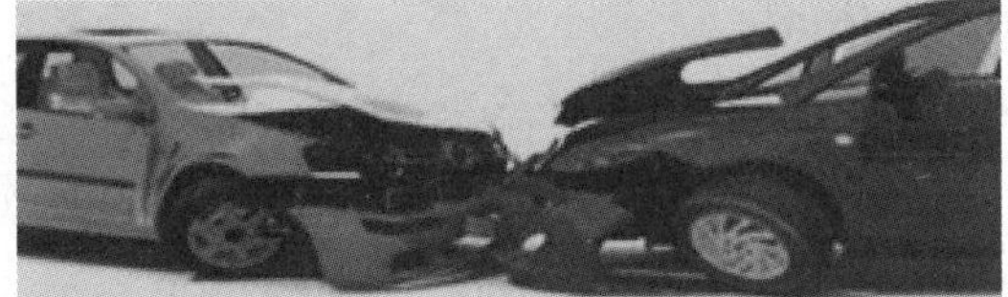

2-1 Trauma Care PPT

Background

Trauma is defined as a variety of injury factors acting on the body, resulting in damage to the structural integrity of the body and dysfunction. Accelerated urbanization and industrialization have led to an alarming increase in the rate of accidents, injuries, crime, and violence. Trauma is an increasingly significant cause to death and disability throughout the world. The main causes of trauma are divided into four categories: mechanical factors, physical factors, chemical factors, and biological factors.

"Every injured individual should have access to—and has a right to—adequate, timely, and effective trauma care that is life or limb saving." Dr. Lin Aung, World Health

Organization Representative to Nepal. Actually, proper first aid treatment can lay a good foundation for the subsequent treatment for various types of trauma, and prevent or mitigate complications, so that patients can be cured successfully. There are four technologies for trauma care: bleeding control, dressing wounds, fracture fixation, and transporting the wounded. In the last task we have learned the life saving technology—CPR; in this task we will learn the four technologies for trauma care.

There are four principles of first aid in trauma care: save life first, treat wound second; serious injuries first, minor injuries second; treat nearby patients first, then treat distant patients; control bleeding first, then dress wounds, fix fracture, and finally delivery the wounded.

2-2 Trauma Care 讲解视频

Bleeding Control

[Objective] To control the bleeding and prevent hemorrhagic shock caused by bleeding.

[Preparation]

Materials preparation: Select the appropriate hemostatic material, such as dressings, bandages, tourniquets, clean clothes and handkerchief.

Patient preparation: position, explanation.

[Common Methods Used to Stop Bleeding]

1. Direct compression to stop bleeding.

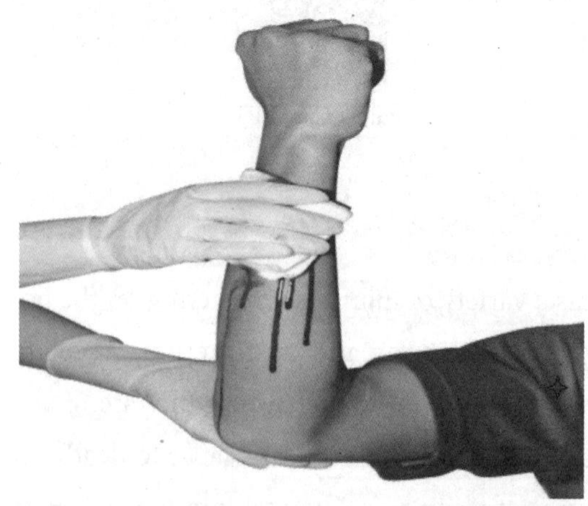

2. Pressure bandage to stop bleeding.

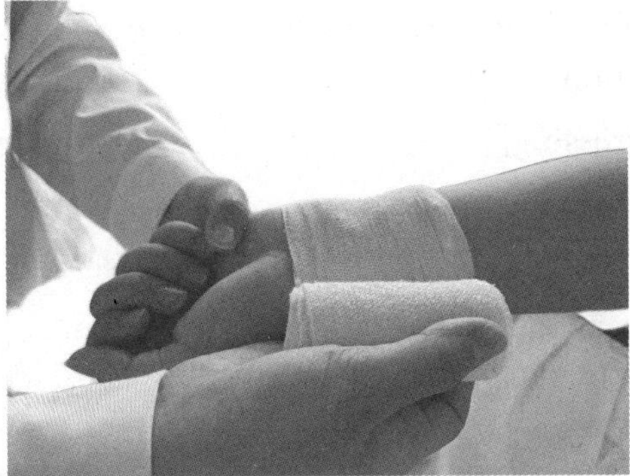

3. Acupressure to stop bleeding.

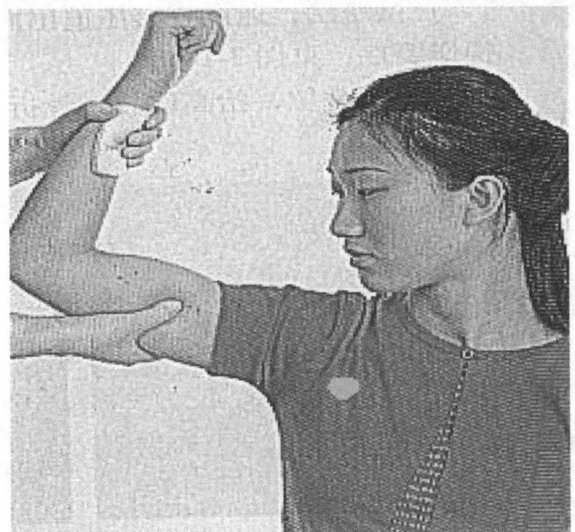

4. Tie up a tourniquet to stop bleeding.

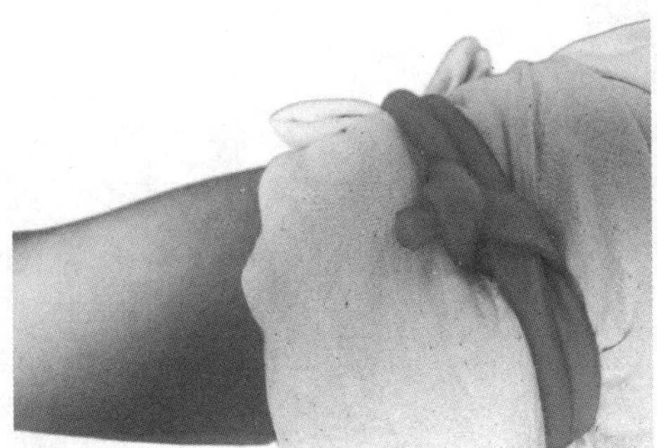

Dressing

[Objective] To control the bleeding, protect the wound from contamination, and fix the fracture.

[Preparation]

Equipment: triangular bandage, bandages, clean cotton, etc.

Patient: position, explanation.

[Common Methods of Dressing]

1. Circular dressing.

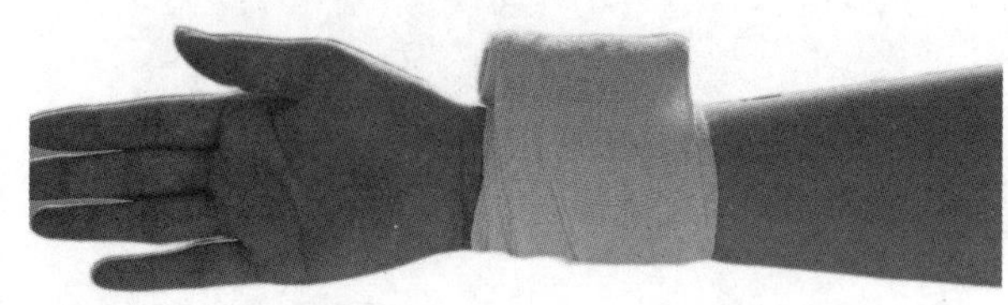

2. Spiral wrap.

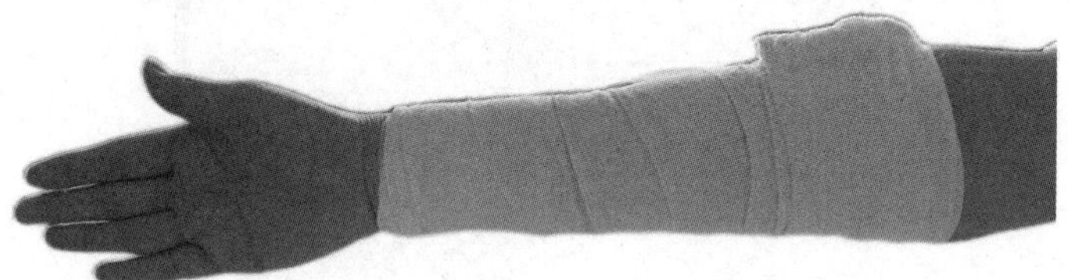

3. Figure of eight bandage.

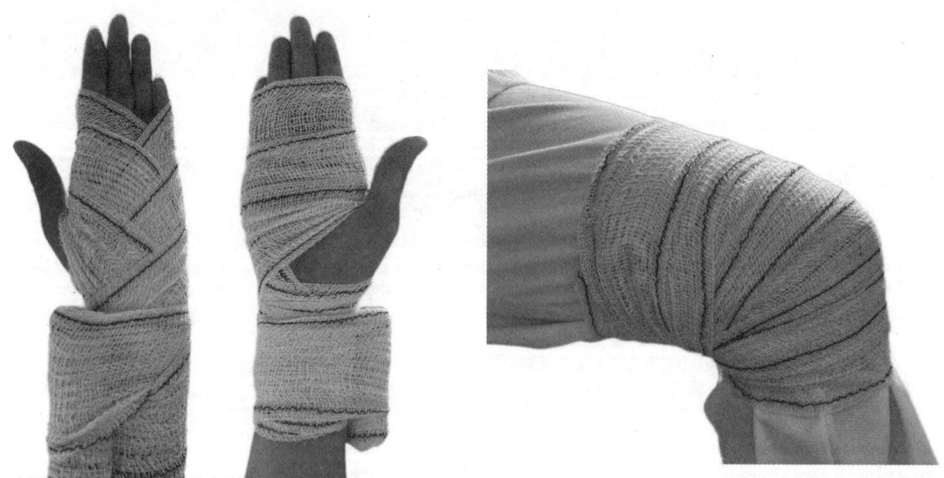

4. Returning bandage.

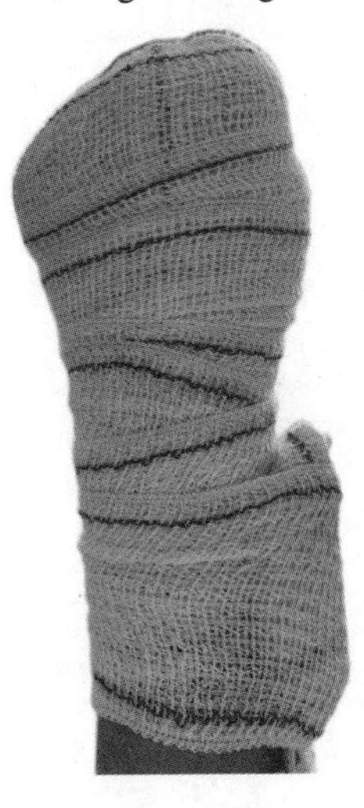

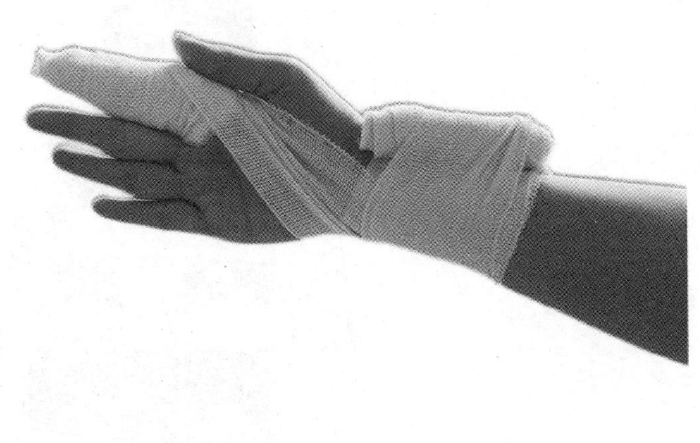

Fixation

[Objective] To restrict activities of the injured parts of the body to relieve pain, and to avoid damage of blood vessel sand nerves caused by displacement of fracture fragments. It helps to controll shock and transfer patients.

[Preparation]

Materials preparation:

First-aid kit: combination of plywood, triangular bandage, bandages, dressings.

Local materials: branches, sticks, cardboards, clothes, towels, handkerchiefs, ties, healthy limb, etc.

Patient preparation: position, explanation.

[Common Methods of Fixation]

1. Fracture fixation with clothes.

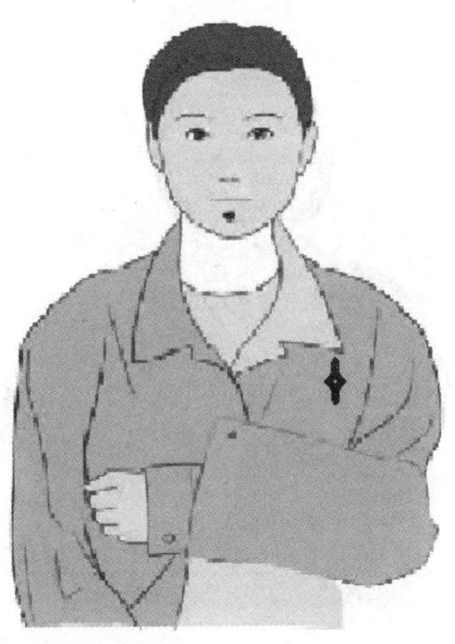

2. Fracture fixation with splint.

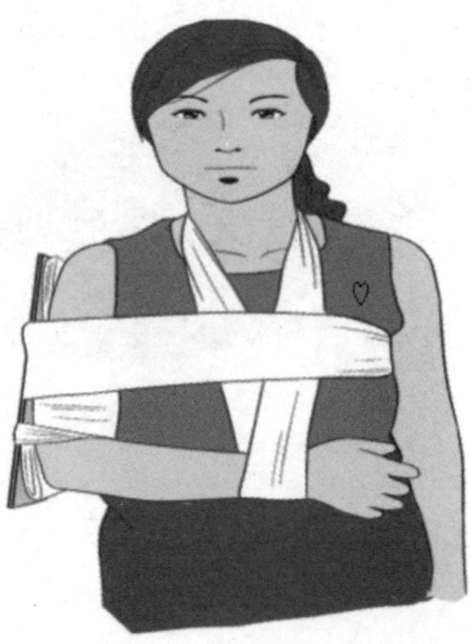

3. Fracture fixation with inflatable splint.

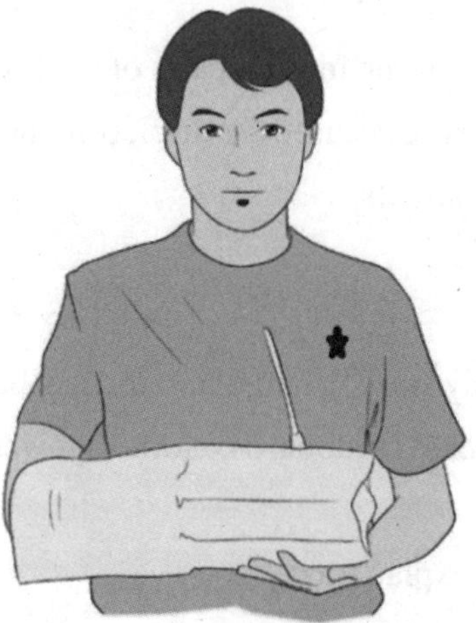

4. Fracture fixation with belt.

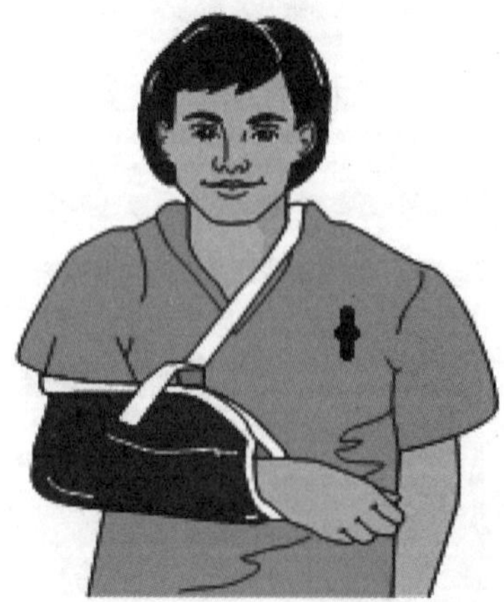

5. Fracture fixation with books.

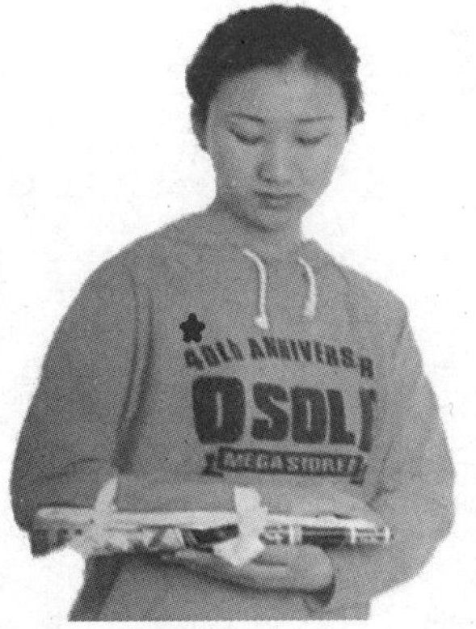

6. Fracture fixation with healthy limb.

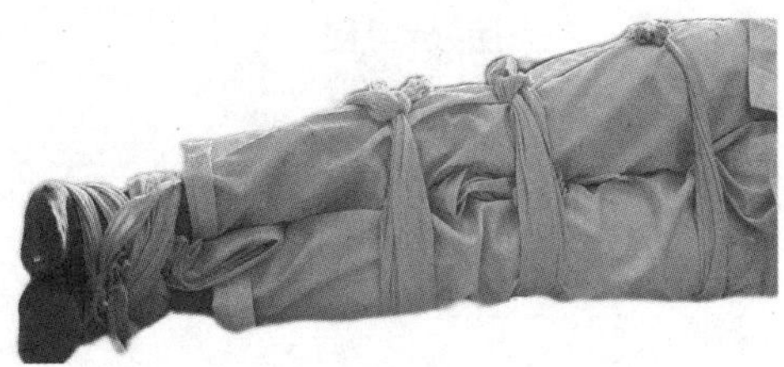

Moving

[Objective] Transfer the wounded out of dangerous environment and alleviate disability.

[Preparation]

Materials preparation: stretcher.

Patient preparation: position, explanation.

[Common Methods of Moving]

1. Manual handling.

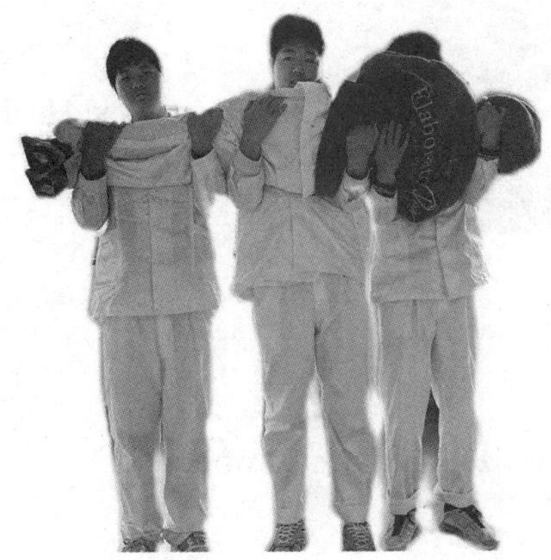

2. Carrying the wounded with a stretcher.

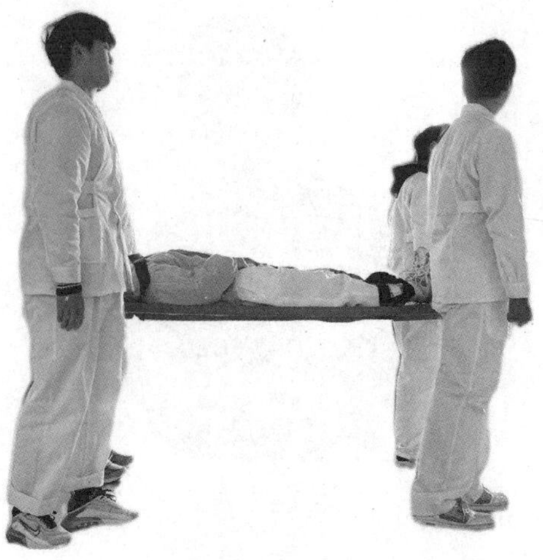

2-3 Trauma Care 操作视频

Procedure

Step 1: Assess environment and determine consciousness.

- The environment is safe. Rescuers should wear gloves and face shields.
- Determine whether the patient could be waked up.

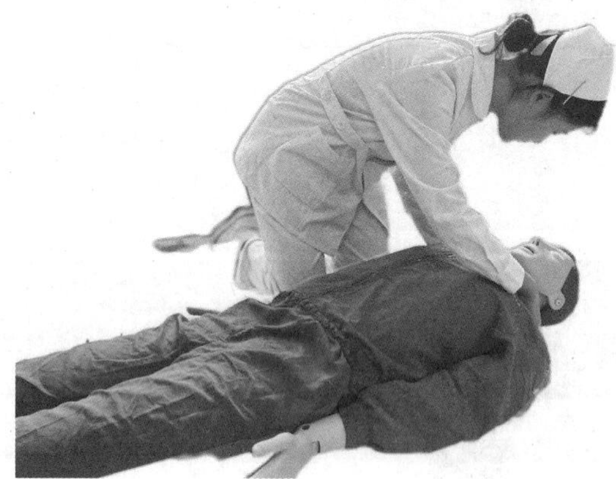

"The environment is safe. Self-protection is ready."

"Hey! Hey! Are you OK?"

Step 2: Initiate EMSS.

- Call 120 the moment you realize the victim is wounded.

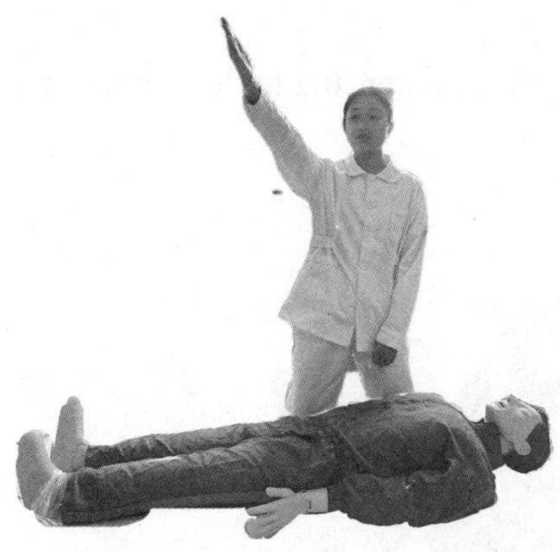

"Help! Help! He needs first aid.
Please call 120 and give me feedback.
Anyone assist me please!"

Step 3: Determine the airway, respiration, and pulse.

- Determine the airway, respiration, and pulse like you do in CPR.
- If the victim is unresponsive, please give the CPR.
- Be alert to the potential for head or neck injury.

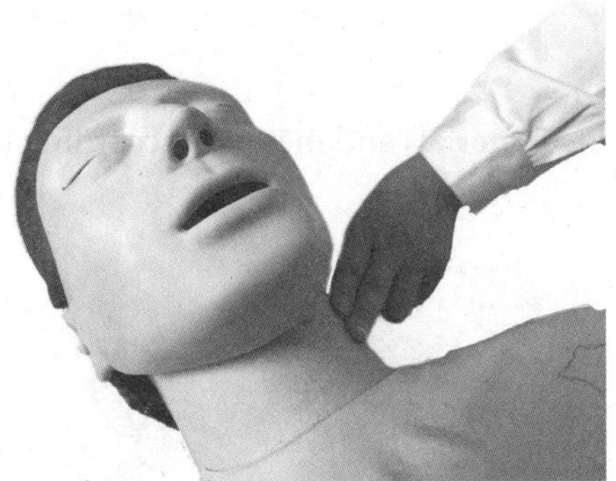

Step 4: Determine injury.

- Determine the injured area in order: neck—thorax—abdomen—back—both arms—both legs. To correctly determine, please assess for 5 to 10 seconds.

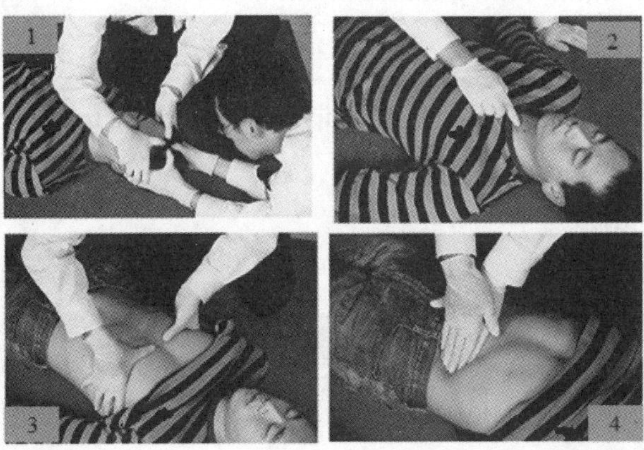

Step 5: Control bleeding.

□ Choose the suitable hemostatic materials and methods according to the condition.

□ Choose the right site to stop bleeding.

□ Looseness is appropriate. Mark it correctly.

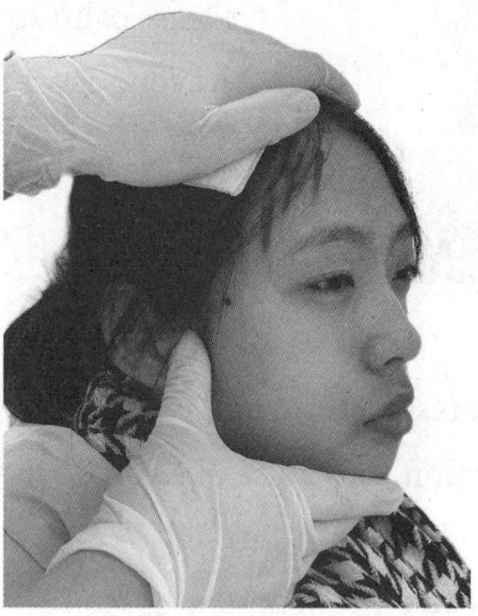

Step 6: Dress.

□ Choose the suitable dressing materials and methods according to the condition.

□ Treat wounds correctly.

□ Looseness is appropriate.

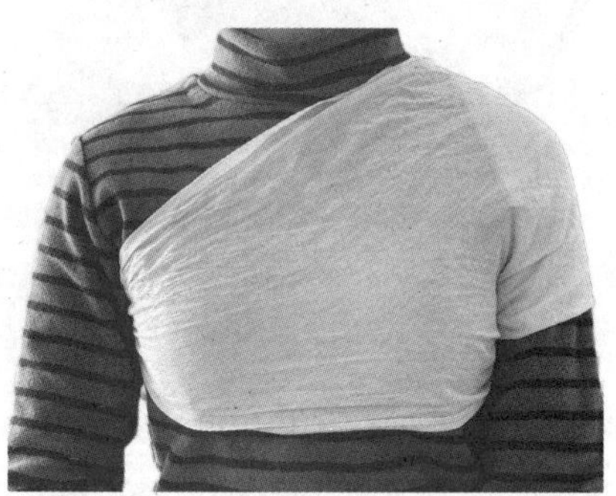

Step 7: Fix.

□ Choose suitable materials and methods for fixation according to the condition.

□ Methods of fixation is correct.

□ Looseness is appropriate.

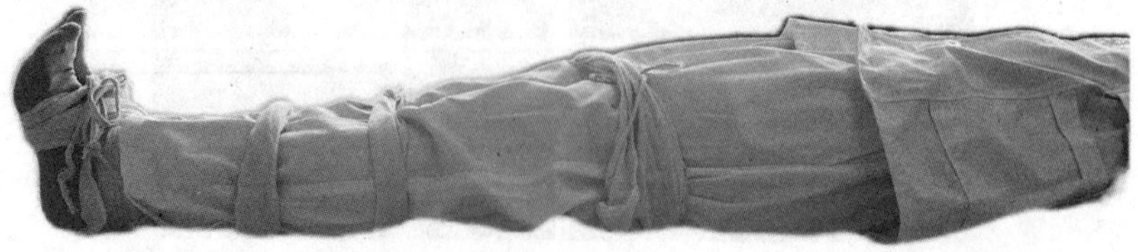

Step 8: Move.

▫ Choose the suitable moving method, especially for the suspected spinal core injury.

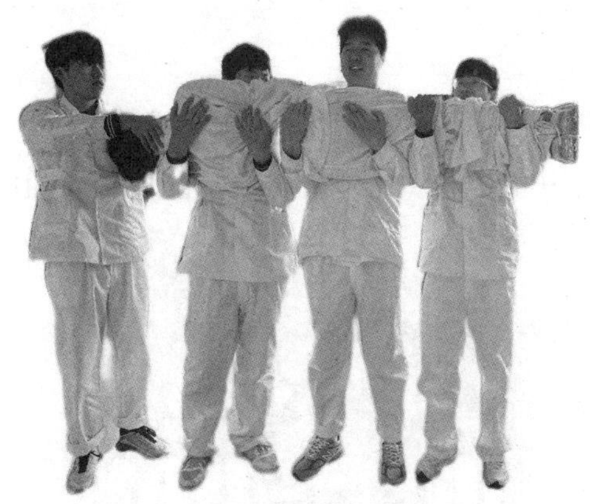

Step 9: Record.

▫ Record the emergency time, process, etc.

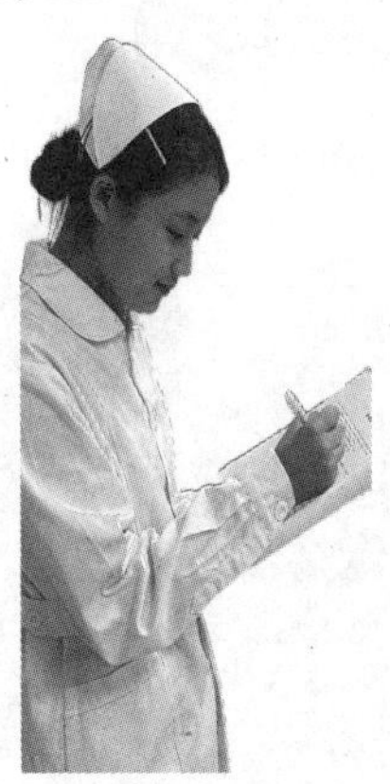

Words and Phrases

cast	石膏	closed/simple fracture	闭合性骨折
external fixation	外固定	open/compound fracture	开放性骨折
internal fixation	内固定	impacted fracture	嵌插型骨折
compartment syndrome	骨筋膜室综合征	greenstick fracture	青枝骨折
fat embolism	脂肪栓塞	comminuted fracture	粉碎性骨折
traction	牵引		

Learning Activities

Part I Choose the best answer for each question.

1. Discuss what kind of first aid you should give in this situation.

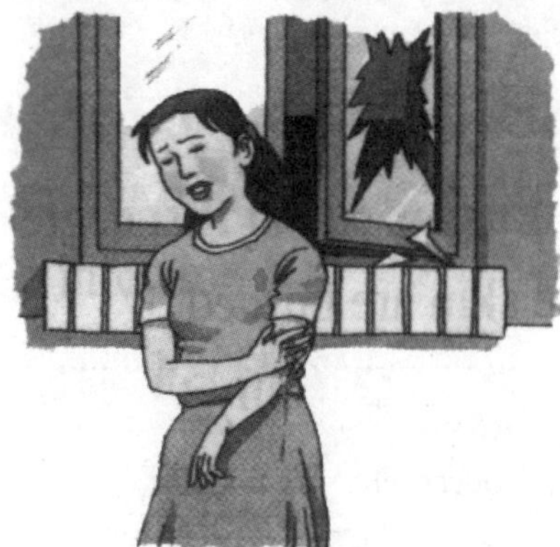

2. Discuss what kind of first aid you should give in this situation.

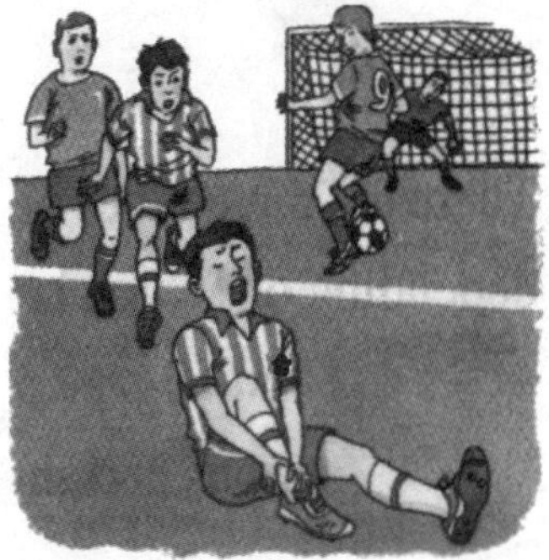

3. Discuss what kind of first aid you should give in this situation.

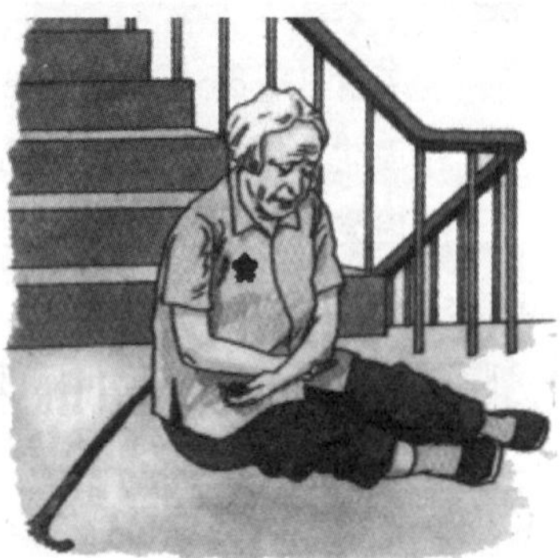

4. Discuss what kind of first aid you should give in this situation.

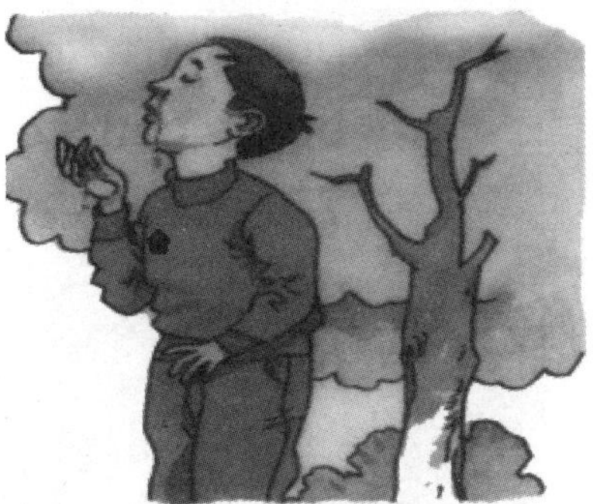

5. Discuss what kind of first aid you should give in this situation.

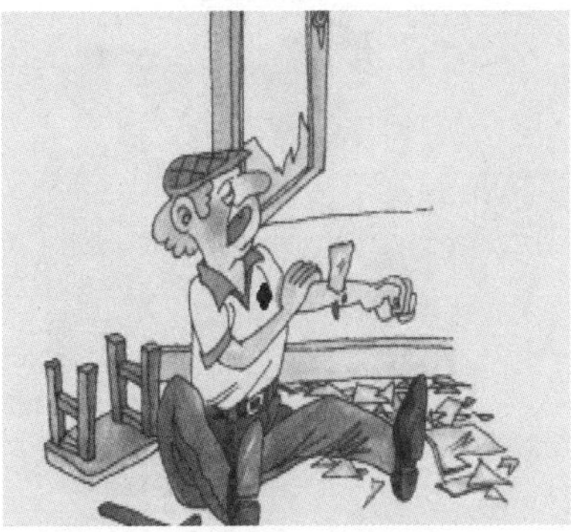

6. Discuss what kind of first aid you should give in this situation.

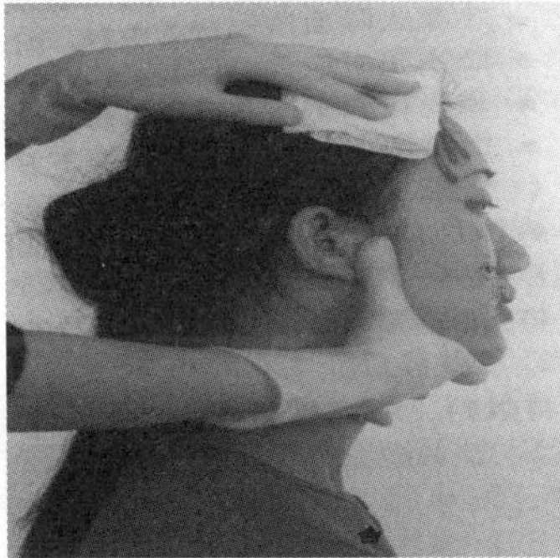

7. Discuss what kind of first aid you should give in this situation.

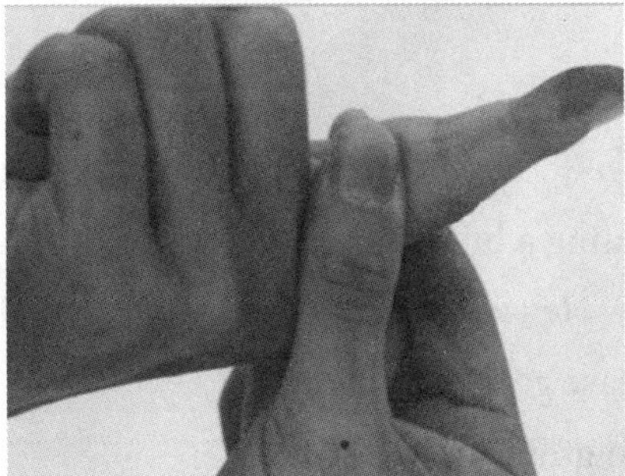

8. Discuss what kind of first aid you should give in this situation.

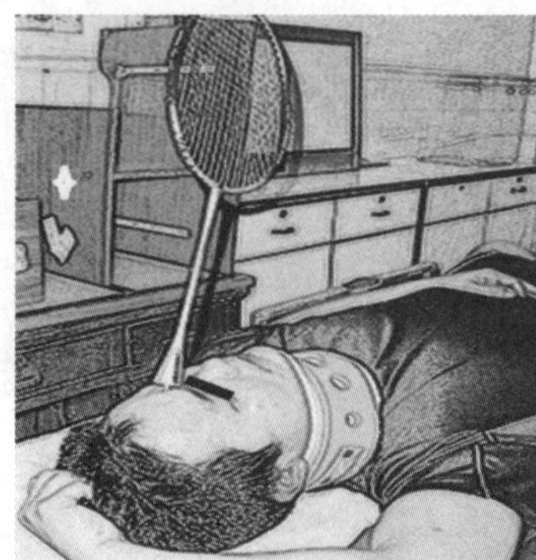

9. Discuss what kind of first aid you should give in this situation.

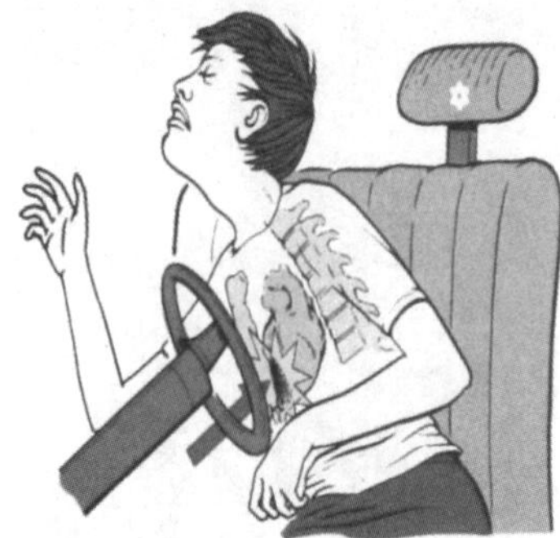

9. Discuss what kind of first aid you should give in this situation.

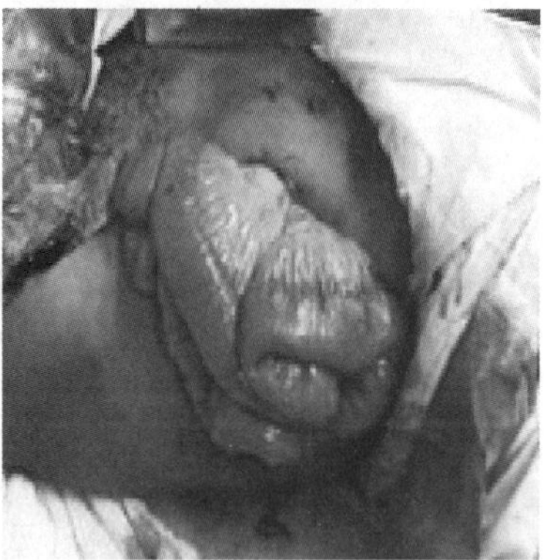

Part II Case study.

Case Scenario

A middle-aged man, riding a bike to go to work, unfortunately collided with a car, and was thrown five meters away. He was severe bleeding of the scalp and left forearm skin, and his left leg was fractured. Please give him the first aid.

Task: Practice trauma care in groups.

（刘桂娟　陈鸿尔）

Scenario Two
Admission

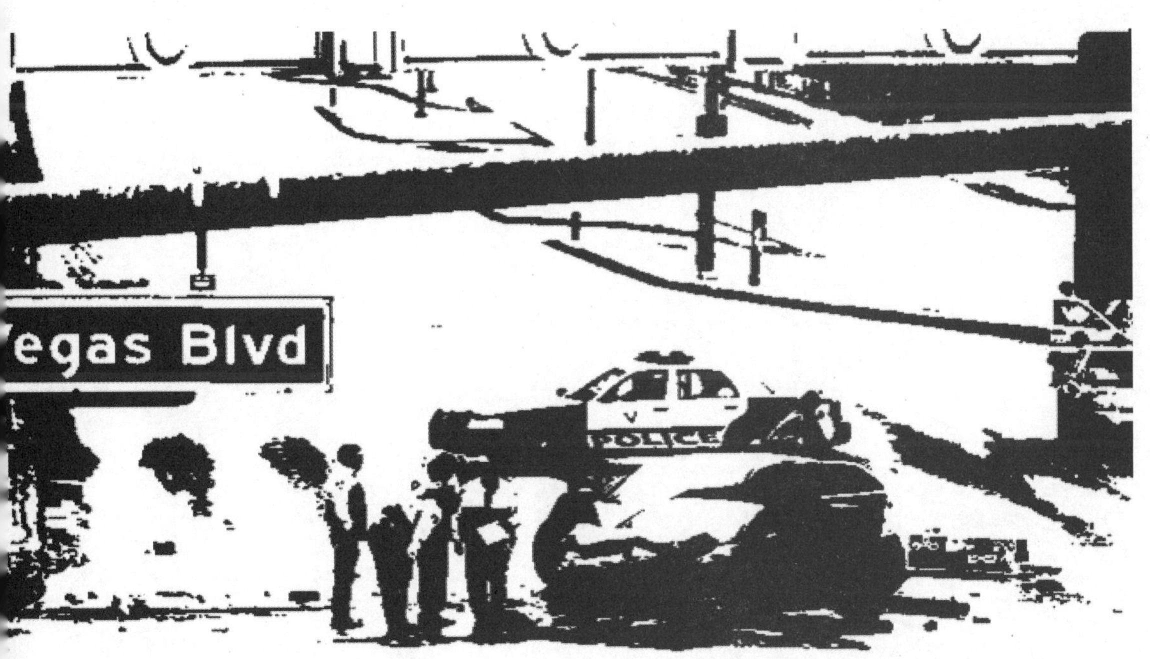

TASK 3

Taking Vital Signs

Learning Outcomes

This task will provide students with opportunities to:

- Assess pulse, respiration, temperature, and blood pressure accurately.
- Explain the physiology of normal regulation of blood pressure, pulse, temperature, and respiration.
- Identify vital signs when vital signs should be taken.
- Record and report vital signs measurement accurately.
- Delegate vital signs measurement to nurse assistants appropriately.

Scenario

Mary, 28-years-old female, had no obvious wound when she was found in the car accident. After she was delivered into the emergency room, she presented with severe headache and intractable vomiting. Physical examination revealed left facial palsy and generalized weakness of the extremities (grade IV/V all extremities) without other localizing signs. She had no known underlying disease and there was no significant family medical history.

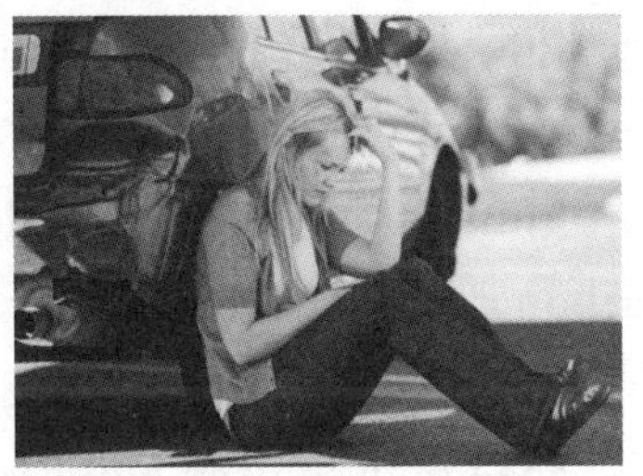

3-1 Taking Vital Signs PPT

Background

The most frequent measurements obtained by health practitioners are those of temperature, blood pressure, pulse, respiratory rate. These measure vital signs which are indicators of the effectiveness of circulatory, respiratory, neural and endocrine body functions. An alteration in vital signs can provide objective evidence of the body's response to physical and psychological stress or changes in physiological function. The unstable vital signs indicated that there are the needs for medical and nursing interventions and monitoring the responses to treatments.

Vital signs assessment is integral to determination of the patient's health status. Careful measurement techniques and knowledge of the normal range in vital signs for a particular patient will ensure more accurate findings and interpretation of those findings.

Temperature is the "hotness" or "coldness" of a substance. The body temperature is the difference between the amount of heat produced by body and the amount of heat lost to the external environment: heat produced−heat lost=body temperature.

Despite extremes in environmental conditions and physical activity, temperature-control mechanisms of humans keep the body's core temperature (temperature of the deep tissues) relatively constant. Surface temperature fluctuates depending on blood flow to the skin and the amount of heat lost to the external environment. The body's tissues and cells function best within a relatively narrow temperature range, with the acceptable from 36 °C to 38 °C.

The pulse is the palpable bounding of blood flow noted at various points on the body. It is an indicator of the fluid wave created by ventricular contraction and therefore of the adequacy of circulatory status.

Human survival depends on the ability of oxygen to reach body cells and for carbon dioxide to be removed from the cells. Respiration is the mechanism which the body uses to exchange gases between the atmosphere and the blood, and the exchange between the blood and the cells. Respiration involves ventilation, diffusion, and perfusion, and can be affected by various factors. These processes can be assessed independently. The rate, depth, and rhythm of ventilator movements indicate the quality and efficiency of ventilation. Diagnostic tests that measure oxygen and carbon dioxide levels in arterial blood offer useful information about both diffusion and perfusion. Analysis of respiratory efficiency requires integrating assessment data from all three interdependent processes. Ventilator adequacy can affect diffusion and perfusion, which in turn will affect ventilation.

Blood pressure is the lateral force on the wall of artery by pulsing blood under pressure from the heart. Systemic or arterial blood pressure, the blood pressure in the system of arteries in the body, is a good indicator of cardiovascular health. Blood flows throughout the circulatory system because of pressure changes. It moves from an area of high pressure to an area of low pressure. The heart's contraction forces blood under high pressure into the aorta. The peak of maximum pressure when ejection occurs is the systolic blood pressure. When the ventricles relax, the blood remaining in the arteries exerts a minimum or diastolic pressure. Diastolic pressure is the minimal

3-2 Taking Vital Signs 讲解视频

pressure exerted against the arterial wall at the times.

Process

[Assessment]

Physical conditions: Choose the appropriate posture according to the measuring location.

Psychosocial status: Assess client's understanding of vital signs measurement related knowledge and client's mental state, and provide basis for health education.

Understanding of treatments and preparations: Make sure the client understand the purpose of vital signs measurement, and recumbent position is comfortable.

[Preparation]

Nurse preparation: Nurses dress neatly, and wash hands.

Supply preparation:treatment plate (glass thermometer, alcohol, watch, sphygmomanometer, stethoscope), record sheet, pen, soft tissue.

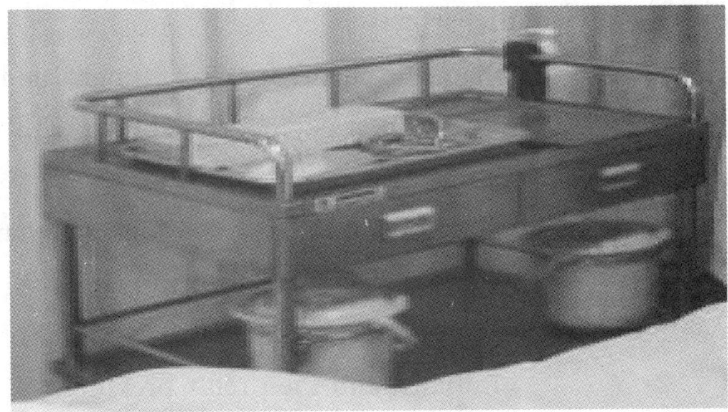

Supplies

3-3 Taking Vital Signs 操作视频

Procedure

Step 1: Oral temperature measurement with glass thermometer.

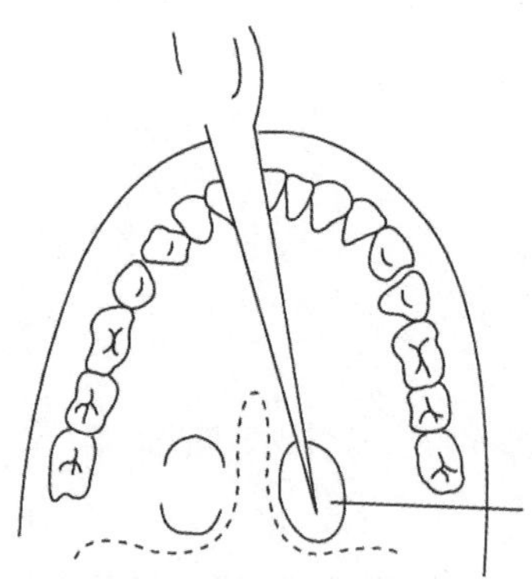

- □ Help the client assume a supine.
- □ Hold the end of glass thermometer with fingertips.
- □ Read mercury level while gently rotating thermometer at eye level. If mercury is above desired level, grasp tip of thermometer securely, stand away from solid objects, and sharply flick wrist downward. Continue shaking until reading is below 35 °C.
- □ Ask the client to open mouth and gently place thermometer under tongue in posterior sublingual pocket lateral to center of low jaw.
- □ Ask the client to hold thermometer with lips closed.
- □ Caution the client against biting down on thermometer.
- □ Leave thermometer in place for 3 minutes and then carefully remove thermometer.
- □ Read mercury level and clean thermometer.
- □ Record.

Step 2: Pulse measurement via radial artery.

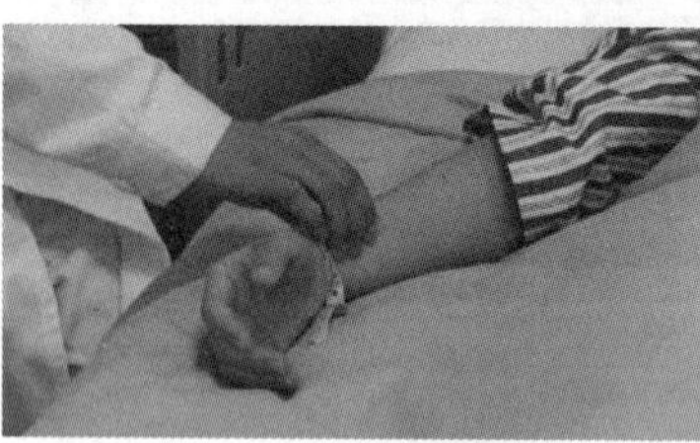

- □ Place the client's forearm straight alongside or across lower chest or upper abdomen with wrist extended straight.
- □ Place tips of the first two fingers of hand over groove along radial side of client's inner wrist.
- □ Lightly compress against radius, obliterate pulse initially, and then relax pressure, so pulse becomes easily palpable.
- □ Determine strength of pulse. Note whether thrust of vessel against fingertips is bounding, strong, weak or thread.
- □ After pulse can be felt, look at watch's second hand and begin to count rate; when second hand hits number on dial, start counting with zero, then one, two and so on.

- If the pulse is regular, count for 30s and multiply total by 2.
- If the pulse is irregular, count for 60s. Assess frequency and pattern of irregular.

Step 3: Respiration measurement.

- While measuring the pulse, observe client's chest undulation.
- If the respiration is regular, count for 30s and multiply total by 2.
- If the respiration is irregular, count for 60s. Assess frequency and pattern of irregular.

Step 4: Measuring blood pressure.

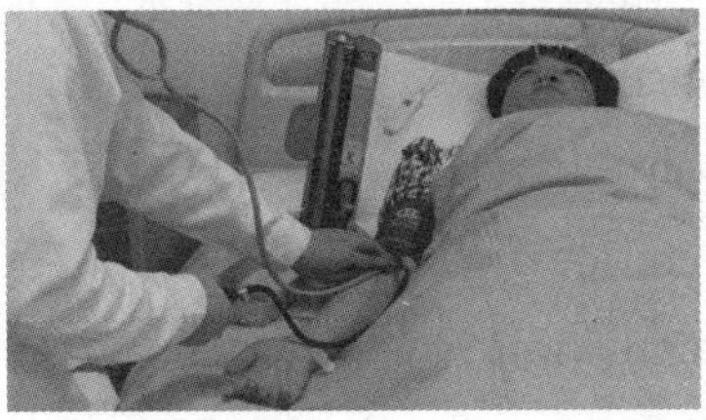

- Expose arm fully by removing constricting clothing. Palpate brachial artery. Position cuff 2.5 cm above site pulsation.
- Apply bladder of cuff above artery by centring arrows marked on cuff over artery. If there are not centre arrows on cuff, estimate the centre of the bladder and place this centre over artery. With cuff fully deflated, wrap cuff evenly and snugly around extremity.
- Position manometer vertically at eye level. Observer should be no farther than 1 m away.
- If you do not know the client's baseline BP, estimate systolic pressure by palpating the artery distal to the cuff with fingertips of one hand while inflating cuff rapidly to pressure 30 mmHg above point at which pulse disappears. Slowly deflate cuff and note point when pulse reappears. Deflate cuff fully and wait 30s.
- Place stethoscope earpieces in ears and be sure sounds are clear, not muffled.
- Relocate brachial artery and place bell or diaphragm chest piece of stethoscope over it. Do not allow chest piece to touch cuff or clothing.
- Close valve of pressure bulb clockwise until tight. Rapidly inflate cuff to 30 mmHg above palpate systolic pressure. Slowly release pressure bulb valve and allow mercury or needle of aneroid manometer gauge to fall at rate of 2—3 mmHg.
- Note point on manometer when first clear sound is heard. The sound will slowly increase in intensity.
- Continue to deflate cuff, and note point at which muffled or dampened sound appears. Listen for 10—20 mmHg after the last sound, and then allow remaining air to escape quickly.
- Remove cuff from extremity unless measurement must be repeated. If this is the first assessment of the client, repeat procedure on other extremity.

- Help the client return to comfortable position and cover upper arm if previously clothed.
- Discuss findings with the client as needed.
- Wash hands and record.

Words and phrases

vital signs	生命体征	ejection	排出物
circulatory	循环的	aorta	主动脉
neural	神经的	systolic pressure	收缩压
endocrine	内分泌的	diastolic pressure	舒张压
integral	完整的	thermometer	体温计
fluctuate	波动	sphygmomanometer	血压计
palpable	明显的；可触知的	stethoscope	听诊器
ventricular contraction	心室收缩	sublingual	舌下的
ventilation	透气	radial pulse	桡动脉
diffusion	扩散	manometer	血压计
perfusion	灌注	relocate	浮动
cardiovascular	心血管的		

Learning Activities

Part I Choose the best answer for each question.

1. The nurse comes to take a woman by wheelchair for a magnetic resonance imaging (MRI) scan of the head and neck. Which of the following observations made by the nurse would require an intervention?________

A. The woman removes her dentures and gives them to her husband.

B. The woman's vital signs are: BP 120/70 mmHg, pulse 80 times/min, respirations 12 times/min, temperature 99 °F (37.3 °C).

C. The woman has a nitroglycerine patch on her right chest area.

D. The woman has red nail polish on her fingers and toes.

2. The nurse has administered sublingual nitroglycerin (nitrostat) to a client complaining of chest pain. Which of the following observations is most important for the nurse to report to the next shift?________

A. The client indicates the need to use the bathroom.

B. Blood pressure has decreased from 140/80 mmhg to 90/60 mmh.

C. Respiratory rate has increased from 16 times/min to 24 times/min.

D. The client indicates that the chest pain has subsided.

3. A male client admitted to hospital due to gastric ulcer. When nurse took his oral temperature, he accidentally bite thermometer. As his nurse, which of the following measures should you take first?________

A. Clear the glass fragments in his mouth.

B. Make the client vomit.

C. Drink lots of milk.

D. Gastric lavage.

4. A female client is suffering from tuberculous meningitis and in a coma. As her nurse, which of the following measures is correct?________

A. When take her oral temperature, nurse should hold her head.

B. Before taking the oral temperature, nurse should take off her false teeth and put it into water.

C. In order to prevent the patient from falling into bed, the restraint should be used.

D. The client's head should be back when inserted nasogastric tube.

5. A dying patient's breathing is very weak. As his/her nurse, what method should you use to measure the patient's breathing?________

A. With ears close to the nose of the patient, listen to his breath.

B. Hand on the patient's chest, count the number of times of the ups and downs.

C. Measure the number of times, and then divided by 4.

D. With a small amount of cotton wire placed in front of the patient's nose, observe the number of cotton yarn swing.

6. Which of the following is not right when the nurse take the pulse of the patient with atrial fibrillation?________

A. Two nurses take the patient's heart rate and patient's pulse independently.

B. Recording mode: heart rate/pulse.

C. Two nurses take the heart rate and pulse at the same time.

D. Put the index and middle fingers in the radial artery.

7. Which of the following nursing observations would indicate to the nurse that a child with epiglottitis is having an early complication of hypoxemia?________

A. Heart rate of 148 beats per minute.

B. Bluish discoloration of the skin.

C. Bluish discoloration around the mouth.

D. Difficulty swallowing.

8. A patient who is receiving hydralazine (Apresoline) q6h has a blood pressure of

90/60 mmHg. Which of the following nursing actions would be most appropriate?________

A. Withhold the medication.

B. Check the urinary output.

C. Administer the medication.

D. Increase the potassium intake.

9. A paitent is diagnosed with lung cancer and undergoes a pneumonectomy. In the immediate postoperative period, which of the following nursing assessments is most important?________

A. Presence of breath sounds bilaterally.

B. Position of the trachea in the sternal notch.

C. Amount and consistency of sputum.

D. Increase in the pulse pressure.

10. The nurse is admitting a paitent to the unit from the postoperative recovery area after abdominal exploratory surgery. After determining the paitent's vital signs, which of the following activities should the nurse perform next?________

A. Position the paitent on her left side, supported with pillows.

B. Check the chart and determine the status of the fluid balance from surgery.

C. Check the paitent's abdominal dressing for any evidence of bleeding.

D. Monitor the incision and pulmonary status for the presence of infection.

Part II Case study.

Case Scenario

A 5-year-old boy comes to hospital because of high fever.

Task: As his primary nurse, please measure the vital signs of the patient.

（郭玲玲　陈巍阳）

TASK 4

Performing an Abdominal Assessment

Learning Outcomes

This task will provide students with opportunities to:

- Memorize usual medical terms about physical assessment.
- Indentify the purpose of physical assessment.
- Define physical assessment techniques.
- Define components of physical assessment.
- Perform an abdominal physical assessment and document the findings.
- Communicate with the client properly while doing physical examination.
- Identify actual/potential health problems stated as nursing diagnosis.
- Perform health education to the client.

Scenario

Mary is a 28-years-old female driver in this severe car crash. The surveillance shows this accident directly caused by her improper drive behavior. She was found without any obvious injury except her forehead slumped over on the wheel in the accident.

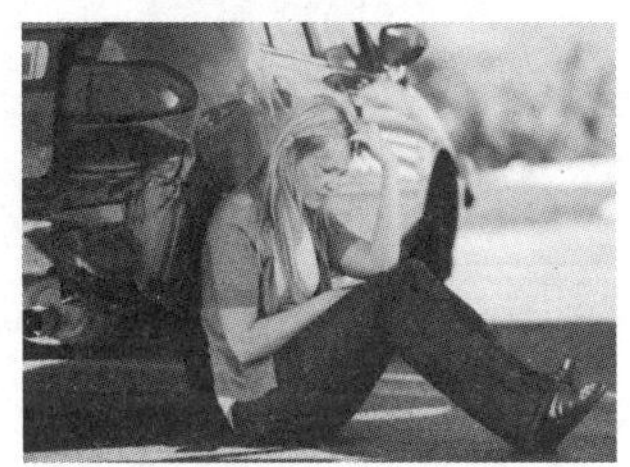

4-1 Performing an Abdominal Assessment PPT

Background

The physical examination is a process by which a medical professional investigates the patient's body for signs of disease and collects the objective data. Where as the health history allows you to see your patient subjectively through her or his eyes, the physical examination now allows you to see your patient objectively through your senses. The four techniques of physical assessment are inspection, palpation, percussion, and auscultation. In this case of the abdominal assessment, auscultation precedes palpation and percussion so as not to alter the bowel sounds. You also need to know normal findings before you can begin to distinguish abnormal ones.

Physical assessment may be either complete or focused. A complete physical assessment includes a general survey, vital signs measurements, assessment of height and weight, and physical examination of all structures, organs, and body systems. Perform it when you are examining a patient for the first time and need to establish a baseline. On the other hand, a focused physical assessment zeros in on the acute problem. You should assess only the parts of the body that relate to that problem.

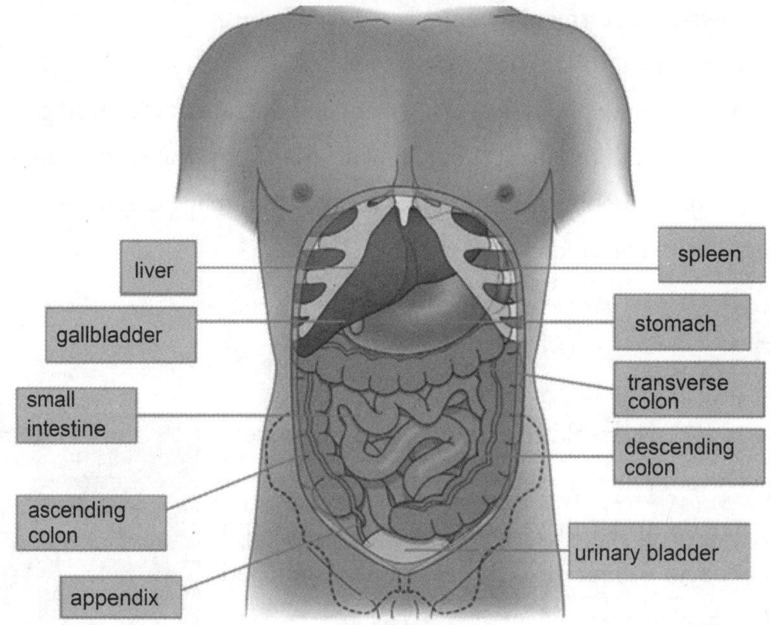

Abdominal Organs and Structures

4-2 Performing an Abdominal Assessment 讲解视频

Process

Now that you have completed the subjective part of your examination, proceed to the objective part. Assessment findings in other body areas can also indicate problems with abdominal organs. So your assessment should begin with a general survey and a head-to-toe scan to detect clues that may indicate an abdominal problem. Use your inspection skills to note nutritional status, emotional status, body habitus, and any changes that might relate to the abdomen. Begin by taking vital signs. Then focus on the abdomen. Begin with inspection and proceed with auscultation, percussion, and palpation. Next, examine each structure separately.

Performing an Abdominal Assessment

Helpful Hints

- Perform the abdominal examination in a warm and private environment.
- Have your patient empty his or her bladder before the examination, so that you do not mistake a full bladder for a mass.
- Ask the patient to lie supine with his or her arms at the sides.
- If your patient tenses his or her muscles when you are palpating the abdomen, place a pillow under his or her knees to relax the abdominal muscles.
- Warm both your stethoscope and your hands before proceeding with the examination, and remember to work from the right side of your patient.
- Once your patient is comfortable, expose the abdomen from the lower thorax to the iliac crests.
- Explain what you will do during the examination.
- Have adequate lighting so that you can visualize the abdomen without difficulty.
- Observe the patient's face for signs of discomfort.
- Perform the examination slowly and avoid quick movements.
- Make sure that your fingernails are short, to prevent injuring the patient during palpation.
- Distract the patient with questions or conversation.
- If your patient complains of pain when you palpate an area, stop, and then palpate that area last.

4-3 Performing an Abdominal Assessment 操作视频

Part I Inspection of the abdomen.

1. Abdomen.

- □ Inspect the abdomen for size, shape, and symmetry. Look at it from different angles. Check color, surface characteristics, contour, and surface movements (respirations, peristalsis, and pulsations). Look for lesions, striae, or scars.

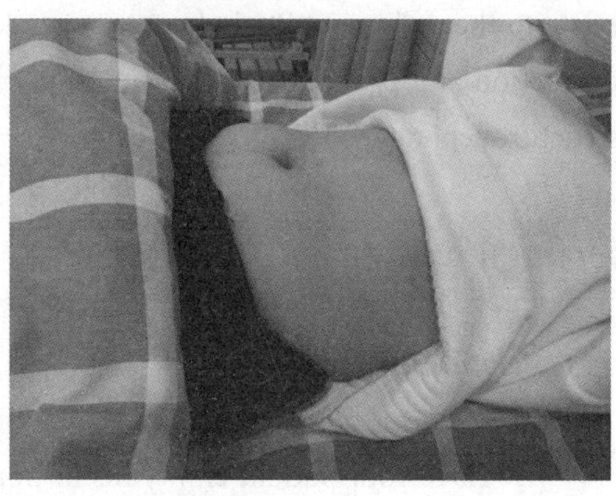

- ▫ Skin color should be consistent with patient's ethnicity. Color may be lighter on abdomen than on other areas of body because of lack of sun exposure. Skin color should be the same throughout the abdomen.
- ▫ Abdominal skin should be intact with no lesions or masses. Striae may be present. If it is new, it should be pink; if old, white or silver. In a pregnant patient, striae and linea nigra may be present.

2. Symmetry.

- ▫ View abdomen from different angles.
- ▫ Abdomen should be symmetrical bilaterally from costal margin to iliac crest, with umbilicus in center.

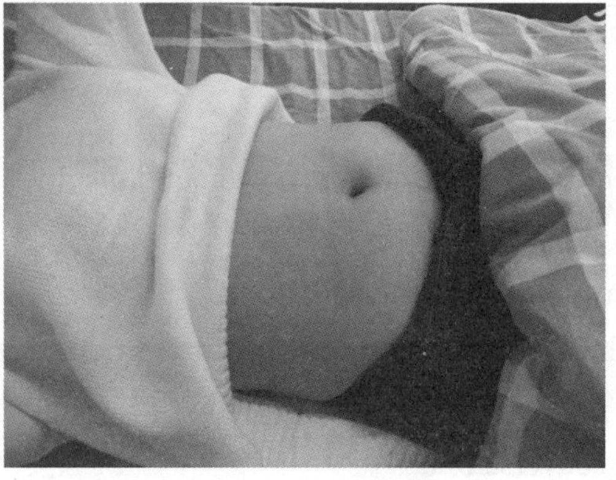

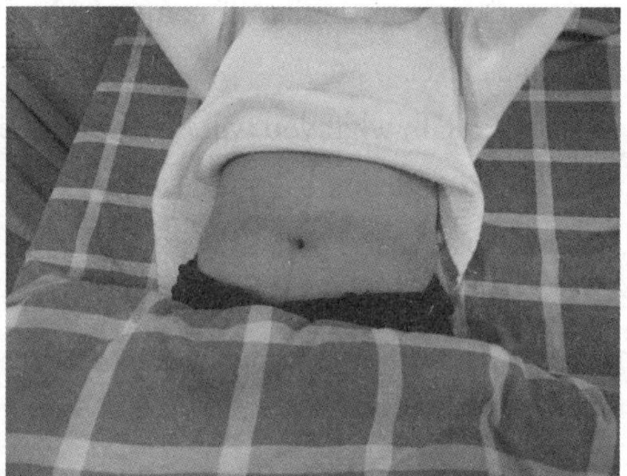

3. Contour and distension.

- ▫ Inspect contour from various angles.
- ▫ No abdominal distension. In average adult, contour should be either flat, round, or scaphoid. A flat contour is seen in a muscular patient who is physically fit. A round or convex contour is normal in infants or toddlers but indicates poor muscle tone or excessive fat deposits in adults. A scaphoid or concave contour may be seen in thin patients of all ages.

4. Surface movements.

- Look for respirations, pulsations, and peristalsis.
- On a thin patient, peristalsis and aortic pulsations may be visible. Women's respirations are more thoracic, whereas men tend to use their abdominal muscles more with breathing.

Part II Auscultation of the abdomen.

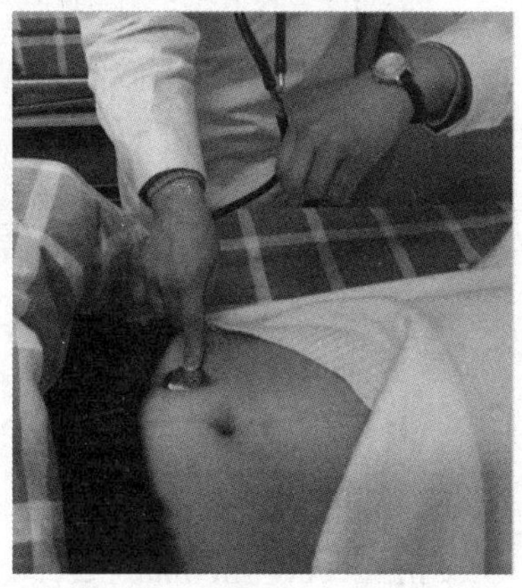

- Begin auscultating the abdomen by placing the warmed diaphragm of the stethoscope gently in one quadrant.
- Proceed in an organized fashion, listening in several areas in all four quadrants.
- Use the diaphragm to listen for bowel sounds, which sound like high-pitched gurgles or clicks that last from one to several seconds. They are assessed to determine bowel motility and peristalsis.

1. Bowel sounds.

- Always auscultate prior to palpation.
- Quadrant off the abdomen with the umbilicus as the midpoint.
- Use the diaphragm portion of the stethoscope to listen for bowel sounds in all four quadrants.
- Listen for at least five minutes before stating patient as absent bowel sounds.
- In an average adult patient, bowel sounds present at a rate of 5—30 clicks/min in each quadrant.

2. Arterial and venous vascular sounds.

- Use the bell portion of the stethoscope to listen for vascular sounds (bruits or venous hums).
- If indicated, listen for bruits over the abdomen at the midline in the epigastric area.
- If indicated, listen for bruits over the renal arteries above the umbilicus to the right and left of the midline in the upper quadrants.
- If indicated, listen for bruits over the iliac arteries below the umbilicus to the right and left of the midline in the lower quadrants.

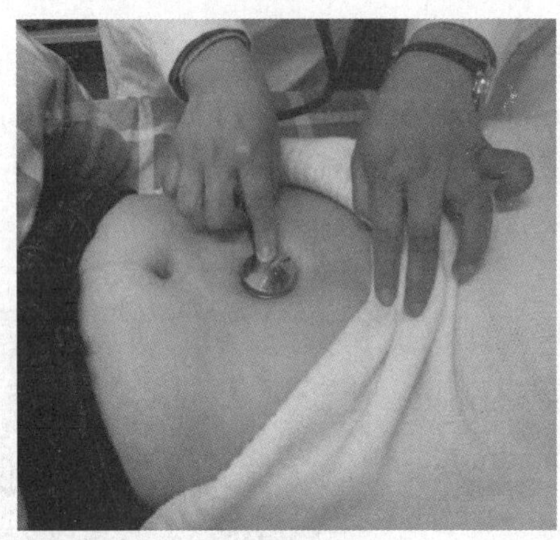

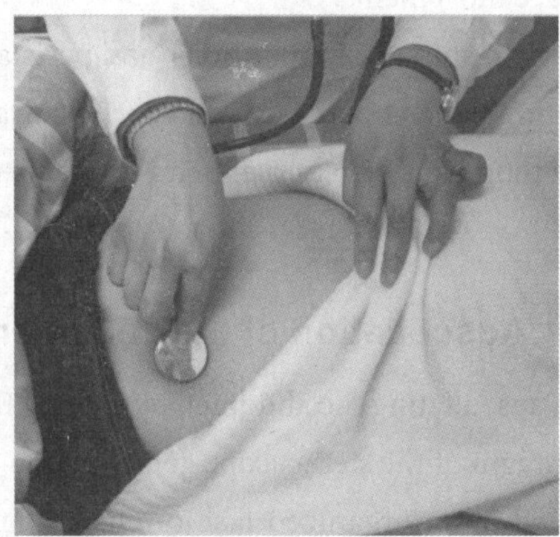

Part III Percussion of the abdomen.

1. Abdomen.

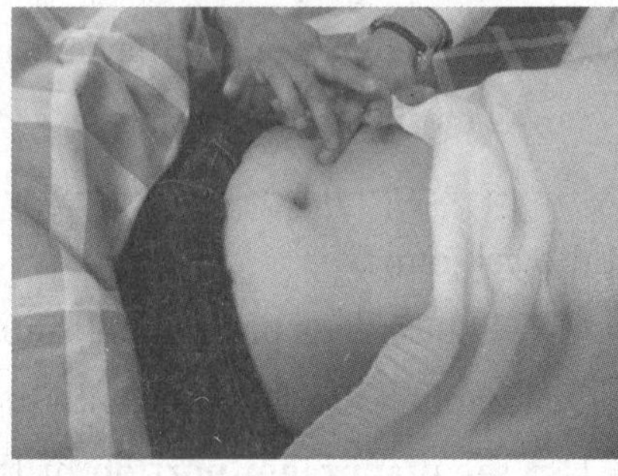

- Use indirect or mediate percussion.
- Percuss the abdomen in all four quadrants, and percuss tender areas last.
- Note areas of dullness and tympany.
- Tympany to dullness, depending on abdominal contents.

2. Liver.

- Use indirect or mediate percussion to determine liver size.
- Locate the upper edge of the liver by percussing downward at the midclavicular line from the fourth intercostal space from resonance to dullness; mark upper border of liver.
- Locate the lower edge of the liver by percussing upward at the midclavicular line from the RLQ from tympany to dullness; mark the lower border of liver.
- Measure the distance between upper and lower marks to obtain liver span.

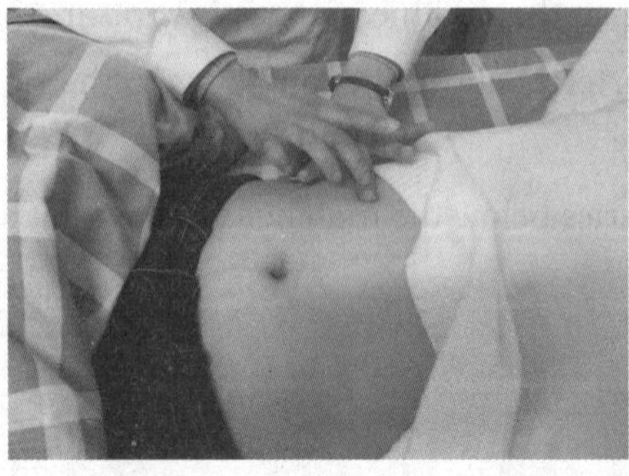

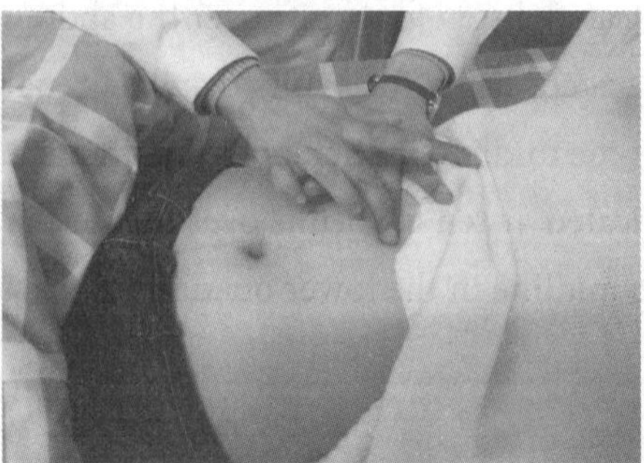

3. Spleen.

□ Identify area of splenic dullness.

□ Position patient on right side, then percuss down the midaxillary line from an area of resonance over the lung to dullness over the spleen.

4. Bladder.

□ If indicated, percuss for bladder dullness at the midline above the symphysis pubis.

□ You should not be able to percuss the bladder above the level of pubic symphysis after the patient has voided.

5. Costovertebral Angle (CVA).

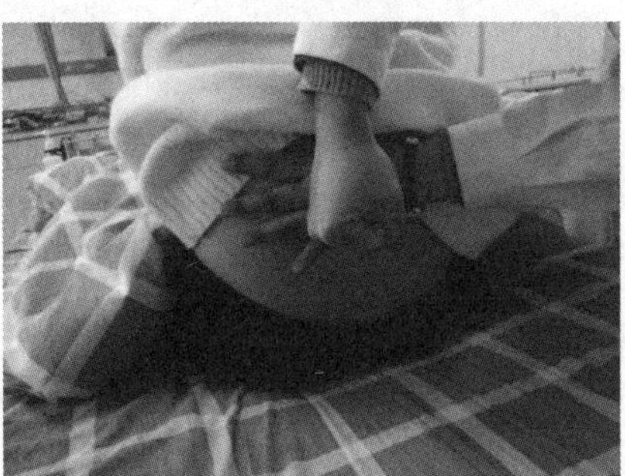

□ Place nondominant hand over kidney.

□ Make a fist with dominant hand and strike nondominant hand.

□ Note any tenderness.

□ Kidney tenderness is assessed at the CVA.

□ No CVA tenderness.

Part IV Palpation of the abdomen.

1. Alert.

□ Do not palpate patients who have had an organ transplant.

□ Do not palpate the abdomen of a child with suspected Wilms' tumor because it may cause the tumor to seed into the abdomen.

2. Light palpation.

□ Lightly palpate about 1/2 inch in each quadrant; palpate painful areas last.

□ Note surface characteristics and areas of tenderness.

3. Deep palpation.

□ Single hand technique: Use dominant hand and palpate greater than 1/2 inch in each quadrant.

□ Bimanual technique: Place dominant hand on abdomen, place nondominant hand on top, and palpate greater than 1/2 inch in each quadrant.

□ Abdomen soft and non tender.

□ No organomegaly or masses, non tender.

4. Palpating the liver.

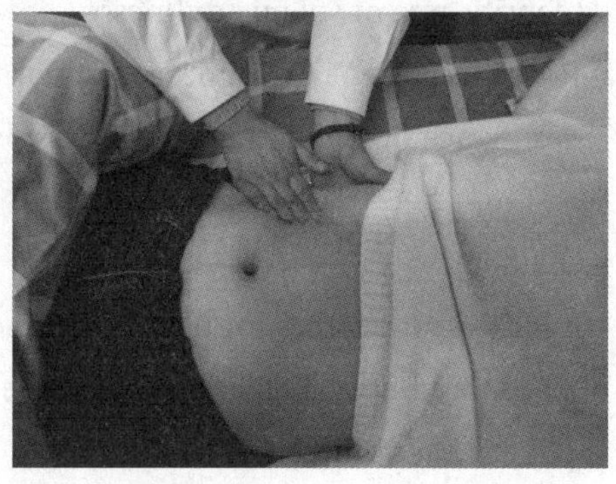

- Stand at the right side of your patient.
- Place the left hand under the patient's back at the CVA, and place the right hand along the costal margin at the right mid clavicular line.
- Have patient take deep breath while you press your right hand in and up, and at the same time with your left hand, press upward to elevate the liver.

5. Palpating the spleen.

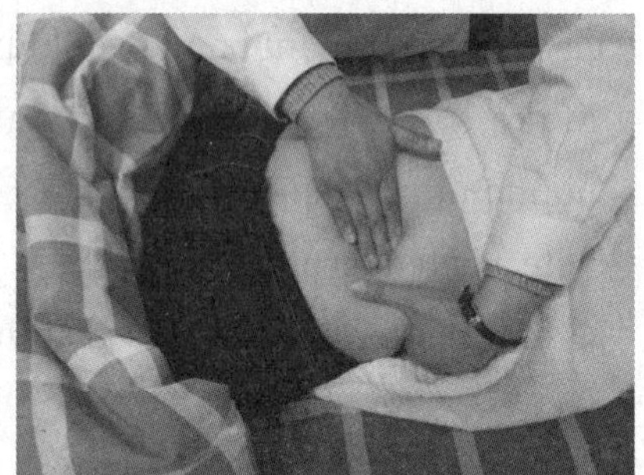

- Stand at the right side of the patient.
- Place right hand under the patient's back at the left CVA, and place left hand along the right costal margin.
- Have the patient take a deep breath while you press inward along the costal margin.

Part V Additional abdominal assessment techniques.

Shifting dullness.

- Have the patient lie supine and percuss the abdomen for dullness and tympany.
- Next have the patient turn on his or her left side and percuss the abdomen.

Words and Phrases

abdomen	腹部	physical examination	身体检查
abdominal	腹部的	objective data	客观资料
liver	肝脏	subjective data	主观资料
spleen	脾脏	inspection	视诊
stomach	胃	palpation	触诊
appendix	阑尾	percussion	叩诊
colon	结肠	auscultation	听诊
urinary bladder	膀胱	nutritional status	营养状况
small intestine	小肠	body habitus	体型

costal margin	肋缘	intercostal space	肋间隙
stethoscope	听诊器	right lower quadrant (RLQ)	右下腹
iliac crests	髂棘	left upper quadrant (LUQ)	左上腹
peristalsis	蠕动波	midaxillary line	腋中线
contour	轮廓	symphysis pubis	耻骨联合
scaphoid	舟状腹	costovertebral angle (CVA)	肋脊角
bruits	杂音	organomegaly	脏器肿大
dullness	浊音	Wilms' tumor	肾母细胞瘤
tympany	鼓音	shifting dullness	移动性浊音
midclavicular line	锁骨中线		

Learning Activities

Part I Choose the best answer for each question.

1. Physical assessments can be either complete or focused. Which situation would warrant a focused physical examination?__________.

A. Student physical examination

B. Pre-employment physical examination

C. Preoperative patient scheduled for hip replacement

D. Patient admitted with chest pain

2. How would you distinguish pain from tenderness?__________.

A. Tenderness occurs with palpation

B. Tenderness is constant

C. Tenderness occurs with or without palpation

D. Tenderness is what the patient tells you it is

3. Johnny's appendix ruptures. What would you expect to hear when auscultating the abdomen?__________.

A. Normal bowel sounds

B. Hypoactive bowel sounds

C. Hyperactive bowel sounds

D. Absent bowel sounds

4. When auscultating the abdomen for bowel sounds, how long should you listen before concluding that bowel sounds are absent?__________.

A. 1 minute

B. 5 minutes

C. 10 minutes

D. 15 minutes

5. When assessing the abdomen, what sequence should the assessment be performed in?_________.

A. Inspection, palpation, percussion, auscultation

B. Inspection, percussion, palpation, auscultation

C. Inspection, auscultation, percussion, palpation

D. Inspection, auscultation, palpation, percussion

6. You are percussing your patient's liver at the right midclavicular line. What is the normal liver span at the right midclavicular line?_________.

A. 2 to 4 cm

B. 4 to 8 cm

C. 6 to 12 cm

D. 8 to 12 cm

7. Tom Johnson, age 56, is admitted to the hospital with the diagnosis of upper GI bleed. Considering his diagnosis, what color would you expect his stool to be?_________.

A. Brown

B. Red

C. Green

D. Black

8. Sam Thomas, age 56, has liver disease. Which area would you most likely hear a venous hum?_________.

A. RUQ

B. RLQ

C. LUQ

D. Left lower quadrant (LLQ)

9. You assess Mr. Brown's abdomen for ascites. Which test is best for assessing abdominal fluid?_________.

A. Shifting dullness

B. Scratch test

C. Iliopsoas test

D. Cullen's sign

10. The nurse is monitoring a patient admitted to the hospital with a diagnosis of appendicitis who is scheduled for surgery in 2 hours. The patient begins to complain of increased abdominal pain and begins to vomit. On assessment, the nurse notes that the abdomen is distended and bowel sounds are diminished. Which is the appropriate nursing

intervention?__________.

A. Notify the physician

B. Administer the prescribed pain medication

C. Call and ask the operating room team to perform the surgery as soon as possible

D. Reposition the patient and apply a heating pad on warm setting to the patient's abdomen

Part II Case study.

Case Scenario

Mrs. Kane is scheduled for a cholecystectomy and has come to the hospital for a preoperative workup. She is a 45-years-old married mother. She has been a part-time accountant for 3 years. As you begin the interview, she says, "Even though I'm a little afraid of surgery, I am glad when my gallbladder is out. It's been causing me a lot of pain." Mrs. Kane is scheduled to have general anesthesia, so a thorough respiratory assessment is necessary.

Task: Now that you have completed subjective data collection, begin collecting objective data by means of the physical examination. Then how to perform respiratory assessment?

（陈　燕　王锡唯）

Scenario Three
Preoperative Nursing

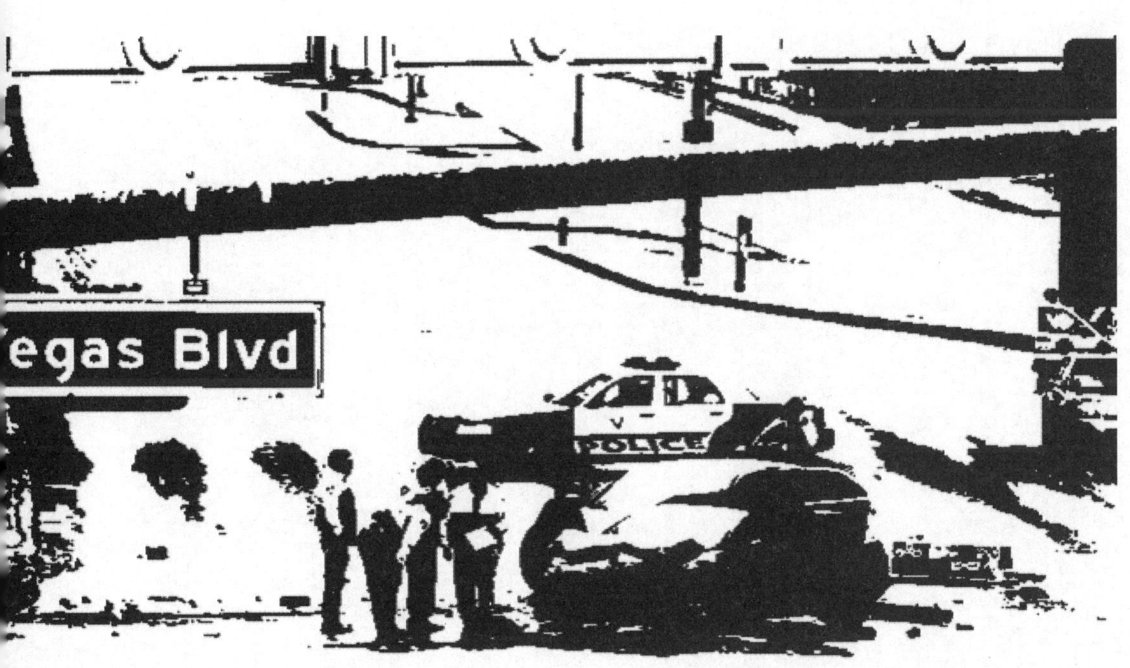

TASK 5

Injections

Learning Outcomes

This task will provide students with opportunities to:

- Explain the preoperative nursing.
- Understand the nursing education in the preoperative nursing.
- Identify injection site according to patients' condition correctly.
- Perform the injection correctly and understand its attention.
- Record and report the documents accurately.
- Cooperate with other health professionals effectively.
- Complete relative nursing practice appropriately.

Scenario

Anne is a 56-years-old driver of SUV. She was taking her 24-week-pregnant daughter Catherine to the hospital for a prenatal physical examination. When the car accident happened, her right calf was stuck in the car and her right arm was bleeding heavily.

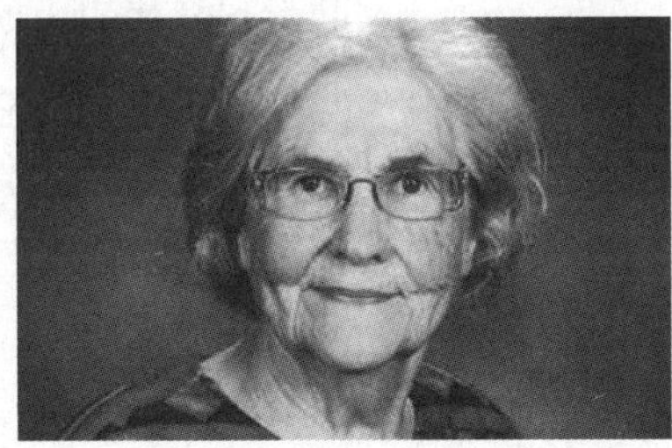

5-1 Injections PPT

Background

Part I

Surgery is an invasive medical procedure performed to diagnose or treat illness or deformity. The surgical procedure involves the interaction of the patient, the surgeon, and the nurse. Perioperative nursing is a specialized area of practice for providing nursing care to the surgical patient, which incorporates the three phases of the surgical experience: preoperative nursing, intraoperative nursing, and postoperative nursing.

Surgery may be performed for any of the following purposes: diagnosis, cure, palliation, prevention, exploration and cosmetic improvement. Surgical procedures are usually categorized according to the purpose (diagnosis, curative, transplant…), risk factor (minor, major), and urgency (elective, urgent, emergency).

The following lists are the preoperative nursing. The nurse should understand and provide the patient and his/her family members with this information.

Patient interview: There would be preoperative interview in advance or on the day of the surgery. First of all, past and current health history , family health history, medications and allergies should be documented. Women should be asked about their menstrual and obstetric history. The nurse should also do physical and psychosocial assessment, for instance, psychological factors related to surgery such as anxiety, fear, as well as social factors such as religious and culture beliefs.

File preparation: Make sure that all required forms have been correctly signed and at present on the chart. The most important one is the informed consent form for the surgical procedure and blood transfusion. The documented physical examination (PE) and the results of laboratory and diagnostic tests such as chest X-ray, ECG, blood chemistry profile, computed tomography (CT) should be on the patient's chart. Lack of these forms may result in a delay or cancellation of the surgery.

Preoperative medications: Preoperative medicines are administered for a variety of reasons. They may promote sedation and amnesia, prevent nausea and vomiting, decrease respiratory and gastrointestinal secretions, and avoid complications after surgery such as antibiotics preventing infections.

Preoperative education: Preoperative education includes the essential information which the patient desires and needs to know before, during, and after the surgery. This information must be tailored to each individual patient and reflect the specific surgery. Patients should receive instruction about a preoperative shower, shave, and enema, food and fluid restrictions. For instance, NPO means no eating of food, drinking (including water) midnight on the night before surgery. Postoperative information includes the need for deep breathing, coughing, and moving. Patients and families should also be told if there will be tube, drainage, monitoring devices or postoperatively special equipment.

Part II

A medication is a substance used in the diagnosis, treatment, cure, relief of prevention of health alternation. The medication may be prescription, non-prescription (over-the-counter) or complementary preparation. In fact, medications are the main treatments patients associate with restoration of health. Because nurses spend more time than other health care workers with patients, they are the most appropriate health care professional to administer and evaluate the effects of medications. Administration of medications is a fundamental part of nursing practice and the nurse draws on knowledge from many life sciences to ensure safe, effective and appropriate medication outcomes for the patient. Regardless of whether patients receive their health care in hospital or at home, the nurse plays an essential role in medication therapy.

In the acute care setting, a nurse spends a great deal of time administering medication to patients. The nurse also ensures that patients are adequately prepared to administer their medications when they leave hospital. In addition, a nurse teaches patients about their medications and their side effects, encourage patients to adhere to their medication regimen and oversees patients self-administration of medications. The nurse evaluates the medications in restoring or maintaining health while providing health education to the patient, family or home health care personnel about the effects and side effects of medications.

5-2 Injections 讲解视频

Process

[Assessment]

Client's Assessment

Selection of the injection site: Assess the injection site skin of the patient to avoid the nerves and blood vessels.

Psychosocial status: Assess the patient's understanding of injection related knowledge and the patient's mental state, and provide basis for health education.

Understanding of treatment and preparation: Make sure the patient understand the purpose of injection. Make sure the patient empty defecate and urinate, and the recumbent position is comfortable.

[Preparation]

Nurse: The nurse dresses neatly, washes hands, and wears a mask.

Equipment: Injection plate (skin

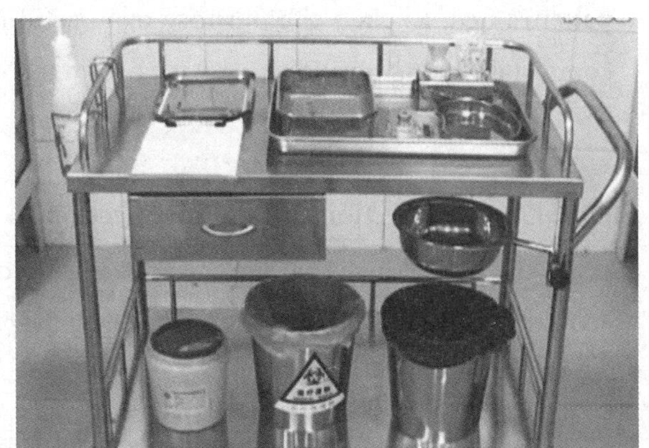

Supplies

disinfectant, sterile swabs, disinfection tourniquet, garbage box), sterilized syringes, infusion cards, sterile patches, disposable venous infusion, solution and drugs.

Environment: Prepare environment according to the principle of sterile practice.

5-3 Injections 操作视频

Procedure

Step 1: Check the doctor's order.

- The order is ready for injection record sheet, which indicates the bed number, name, drug name, dosage, concentration, usage and time. Check the name of the drag name, concentration, clarity, presence of particles, suspension, etc.

Step 2: Suction liquid correctly.

- Check again. Check the quality of the injection drug and the signature. Then suction liquid.
- After that, finish all the supplies, wash hands, and take the supplies to patient.

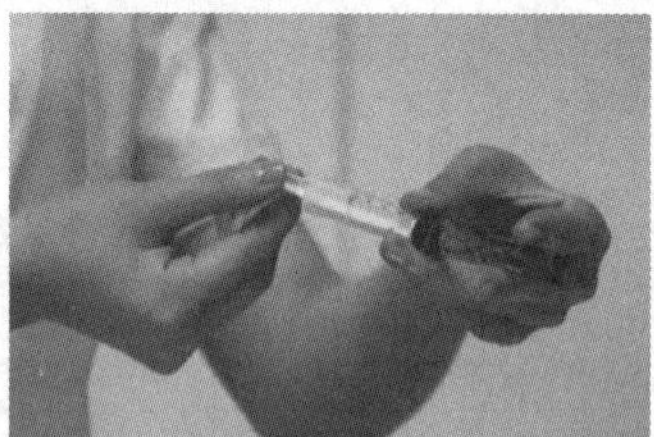

Suction Liquid

Step 3: Check and explain.

- Check the injection information according to doctor's order again, and push it to the patient's bed. Explain the purpose of injection, injection site, and assist the patient to comfortable lying position.

Step 4: Choose injection site and disinfection.

- Assess the skin of injection site (no scar, no scleroma, avoid blood vessels and nerves).
- Sterile the skin of the injection site (centered on the puncture site, more than 5 cm in diameter).

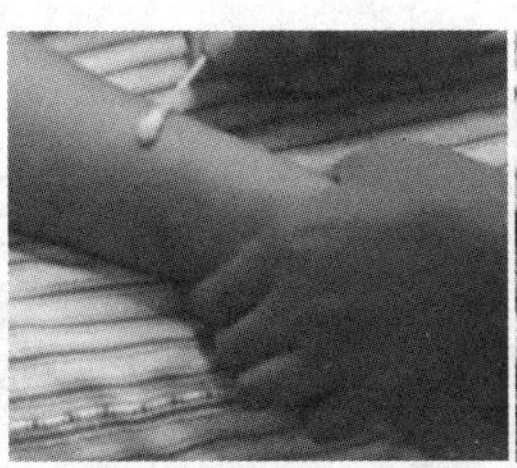
Intradermal Injection Site

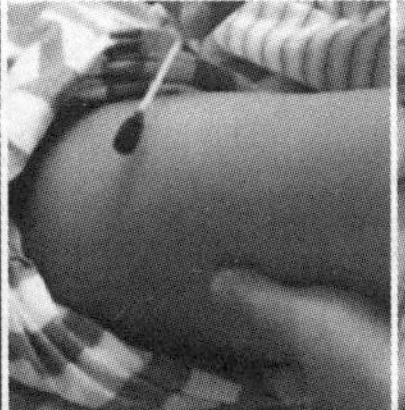
Subcutaneous Injection Site

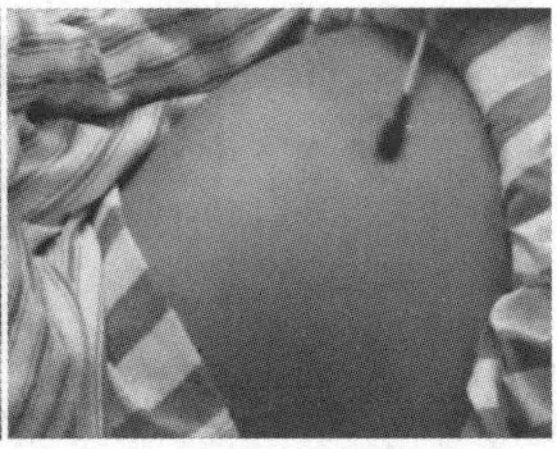
Intramuscular Injection Site

Step 5: Exhaust the air for the second time and give injection.

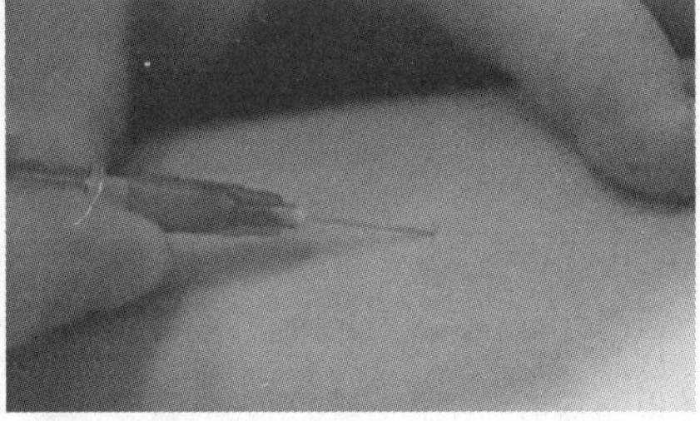
Intradermal Injection

- Intradermal injection: With non-dominate hand, stretch skin over site with forefinger or thumb. With needle almost against the patient's skin, insert it slowly at less than 5 degree angle until resistance is felt. Then advance needle through epidermis to approximately 3 mm below skin surface. Inject medications slowly. Normally, resistance is felt. If not, needle is too deep; remove and begin again.

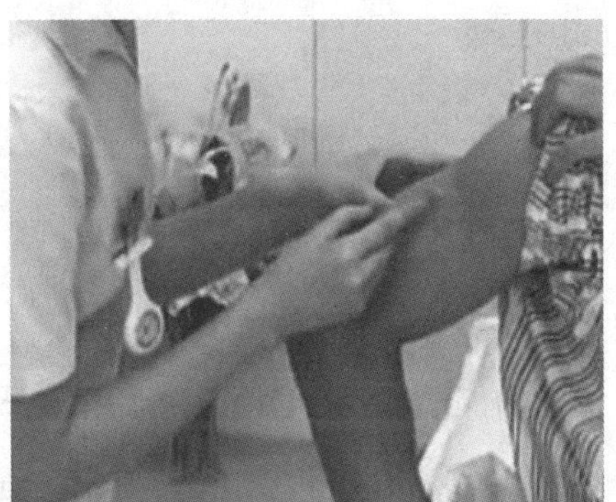
Subcutaneous Injection

- Subcutaneous injection: Spread skin tightly across injection site or pinch skin with non-dominant hand. Inject needle quickly and firmly at 45—90 degree angle. Then release skin, if pinched. For obese patient, pinch skin at site and inject needle at 90 degree angle below tissue fold. After needle enters site, grasp lower end of syringe barrel with non-dominant hand. Move dominant hand to end of plunge. Avoid moving syringe while slowly pulling back on plunge to aspirate drug. If blood appears in syringe, remove needle, discard medication and syringe, and repeat procedure. Inject medication slowly, about 10 seconds, smoothly, and steadily.

Step 6: Record, clear up, and observe.

- Record injection time, drug, dosage, drop on the injection card, assist the patient to comfortable lying position, and tell the matters of attention before you leave the ward. After injection, observe the patient's reaction, and ask the help if the patient has any discomfort.

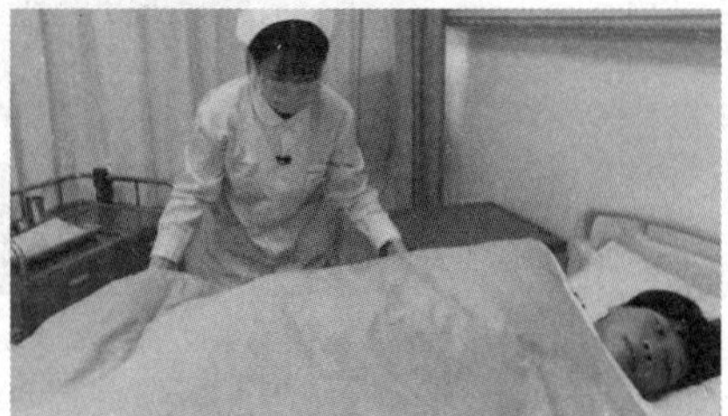

Warning

Words and Phrases

perioperative nursing	围手术期护理	injection	注射
palliation	减轻（痛苦）	substance	物质
curative	治疗性的	over-the-counter	非处方药
allergies	过敏	scleroma	硬结
sedation	镇静	intradermal	皮内的
amnesia	麻醉	subcutaneous	皮下的
enema	灌肠剂	intramuscular	肌内的
drainage	引流管		

Learning Activities

Part I Choose the best answer for each question.

1. A toddler admitted with an elevated blood lead level is to be treated with intramuscular (IM) injections of calcium disodium edetate (Calcium EDTA) and dimercaprol (BAL). Which of the following nursing actions should have the highest priority? _________

A. Keep a tongue blade at the bedside.

B. Encourage the child to participate in play therapy.

C. Apply cool soaks to the injection site.

D. Rotate the injection sites.

2. An 18-month-old baby is brought by her father to the well-baby clinic for a routine immunization. Just before the nurse gives the injection, the baby begins to cry. Which of the following comments by the nurse is the most appropriate? _________

A. "Don't cry. It will be better if you try to behave."

B. "I know you are frightened. It will be over with soon."

C. "A big girl like you shouldn't cry. It's only going to hurt a little."

D. "Please stop crying. There is nothing to be afraid of."

3. The nurse is preparing a client for a skin biopsy. Which of the following client's statements should be reported to the physician by the nurse? _________

A. "I've been taking aspirin for my sore knees."

B. "Using lotion has helped my dry skin."

C. "I went to the tanning salon yesterday."

D. "I had a big breakfast this morning."

4. The nurse is teaching a client how to perform self-monitoring blood glucose (SMBG) by using a blood glucose monitor. Which of the following actions, if performed by the client, indicates to the nurse the need for further teaching? _________

A. The client lets her hand dangle before sticking her finger with the lancet.

B. The client sticks her finger on the side of the distal phalanx.

C. The client touches the strip with a large drop of blood hanging from her fingertip.

D. The client milks her finger after sticking it.

5. A client who is receiving hydralazine (Apresoline) q6h has a blood pressure of 90/60 mmHg. Which of the following nursing actions would be most appropriate? _________

A. Withhold the medication.

B. Check the urinary output.

C. Administer the medication.

D. Increase the potassium intake.

6. A 34-year-old multipara comes to the prenatal clinic during her fifth month of pregnancy. The client complains to the nurse that her breasts are sensitive and sore. Which of the following suggestions made by the nurse is best? _________

A. Apply warm compresses to your breasts and take two aspirin as needed.

B. Massage your breasts with lotion and wear loose-fitting clothing.

C. Apply cold compresses to your breasts and wear a well-fitting, supportive bra.

D. Take a diuretic once a day and avoid touching your breasts.

7. Two days after admission, a client's sputum culture is reported as positive for tuberculosis. While awaiting orders from the physician, the nurse should _________

A. initiate measures to transfer the client to a tuberculosis unit.

B. institute measures to initiate airborne precautions.

C. arrange for all of the client's personal effects to be decontaminated.

D. notify the client's family that they have been exposed to a contagious disease.

8. The nurse is caring for a 17-year-old married male scheduled for a hernia repair. The nurse administers meperidine hydrochloride (Demerol) 50 mg and hydroxyzine pamoate (Vistaril) 25 mg IM. Thirty minutes later, the nurse discovers that the informed consent is unsigned. Which of the following actions taken by the nurse is best? ________

A. Cancel the surgery.

B. Ask the client to sign the informed consent.

C. Notify the physician.

D. Ask the client's mother to sign the informed consent.

9. The physician orders naproxen sodium (Anaprox) 250 mg enteric-coated tablets PO bid for a 45-year-old man. Which response, if made by the client, would indicate that the nurse's teaching about the medication has been effective? ________

A. "I can join my wife in a glass of wine with our dinner when we eat in a restaurant."

B. "I should avoid milk and dairy products when I take this pill."

C. "I should call my doctor if my stool turn very dark."

D. "I don't like to take pills so I will crush the pill and add it to some applesauce."

10. A child admitted with failure to thrive has just had a positive sweat test. Which of the following changes in the child's plan of care would the nurse anticipate initially? ______

A. Administration of replacement enzymes.

B. Administration of oxygen.

C. A salt-restricted diet.

D. Initiating intravenous therapy.

11. While teaching the client about the importance of prenatal vitamins, the nurse should tell the client to take the vitamins ________

A. with orange juice at bedtime.

B. at breakfast with coffee.

C. with milk at lunch.

D. with water at dinner.

12. The physician prescribes sucralfate (Carafate) 1 gm PO tid and 2 Maalox tablets tid for a 50-year-old man in the outpatient clinic. The client asks the nurse the time to take these medications. The nurse should advise the man to take ________

A. the Carafate and the Maalox 1 hour ac.

B. the Maalox 1 hour ac and the Carafate 1 hour pc.

C. the Carafate and the Maalox 2 hours pc and hs.

D. the Carafate 1 hour ac and the Maalox 1 hour pc.

13. A client develops severe, crushing chest pain radiating to the left shoulder and arm. Which of the following PRN medications should the nurse administer? _________

A. Diazepam (Valium) PO.

B. Meperidine (Demerol) IM.

C. Morphine sulfate IV.

D. Nitroglycerine (Nitrostat) SL.

14. A client comes to the nurse's station for her antipsychotic medication. The nurse notes that the client has torticollis, an arched back, and rapid movement of the eyes. Which of the following action should the nurse take first? _________

A. Determine what other medications the patient is taking.

B. Perform a neurological assessment.

C. Administer haloperidol decanoate (Haldol D) IM stat.

D. Administer the PRN trihexyphenidyl (Artane) IM immediately.

15. The home health nurse is performing a follow-up visit for a 76-year-old man receiving isoniazid (INH) 200 mg every day for 6 months. Which of the following statements made by the client would be most concerned by the nurse? _________

A. "I have blurred vision at times."

B. "My legs and knees hurt."

C. "My hands and feet tingle."

D. "I think I had a migraine yesterday."

Part II Case study.

Case Scenario

Jenny, 70-year-old female, came to outpatient because of high fever for a whole day, PE: T 39.8 °C, P 116 bpm, R 28 times/min, Bp 132/78 mmHg. Diagnosis: pneumonia. The doctor advised the patient to be hospitalized and prescribed the doctor's order: 800U penicillin IM.

Task:(1) You are the primary nurse of the patient. What is the first thing you should do before intramuscular?

(2) What should you pay attention to when you perform the intramuscular for the patient?

（郭玲玲　林　凯）

TASK 6

Peripheral Intravenous Infusion

Learning Outcomes

This task will provide students with opportunities to:

- Identify solution and infusion site according to patients' condition correctly.
- Perform intravenous infusion correctly and deal with failure of infusion.
- Cooperate and communicate with other health professionals effectively.
- Complete relative nursing documents appropriately.

Scenario

David was walking across the road after shopping for groceries when the accident happened. It occurred so suddenly that he was unable to step aside. He was heavily crashed by Mary's car and bounced five meters off. Someone called 911 and someone else yelled into the store for help. His pulse and breath were absent immediately. MRI showed he got a hepatic rupture. He got an emergency surgery immediately to save his life.

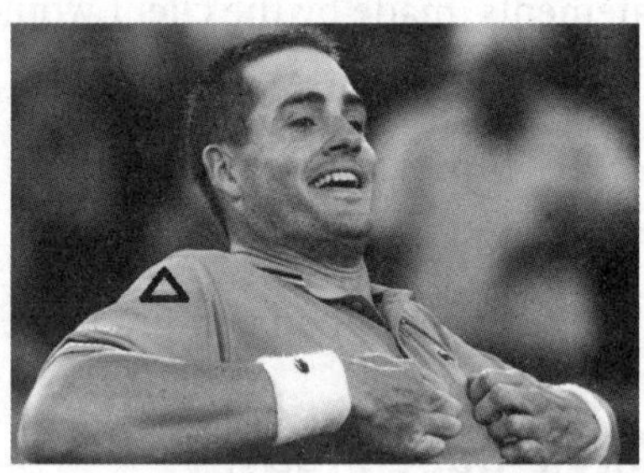

6-1 Peripheral Intravenous Infusion PPT

Background

Fluid, electrolyte, and acid-base balances within the body are necessary to maintain health and function in all body systems. These balances are maintained by the intake and output of water and electrolytes and regulation by the renal and pulmonary systems. Imbalances may result from many factors, including illnesses, altered fluid intake, or prolonged episodes of vomiting or diarrhea. Acid-base balance is necessary for many physiological processes, and imbalance can alter respiration, metabolism, and the function of the central nervous system. Intravenous infusion (IV) is one of the important measures to correct the body's fluid, electrolyte, and acid-base balance.

IV fluid administration is defined as the infusion of liquid substances directly into a vein. The goal is to maintain fluid, electrolyte, and acid-base balance. Intravenous fluid therapy must be closely regulated because of continual changes in the patient's fluid, electrolyte, and acid-base balance.

When IV fluid administration is required, the nurse must know the correct ordered solution, the equipment needed, the procedures required to initiate an infusion, how to regulate the infusion rate and maintain the system, how to identify and deal with problems, and how to discontinue the infusion if necessary.

Types of solutions: Many prepared IV solutions are available for use. Intravenous solutions are either isotonic, hypotonic or hypertonic(see Table 6-1). Isotonic solutions are those that have the same effective osmolality as body fluids. Hypotonic solutions are those that have en effective osmolality less than body fluids. Hypertonic solutions are those that have an effective osmolality greater than body fluids.

Table 6-1 Intravenous Solutions

Solution	Concentration	Other names
Glucose (=dextrose) in water solution		
Glucose 5% in water	Isotonic	G5W(D5W)
Glucose 10% in water	Hypertonic	G10W(D10W)
Saline solutions		
0.45% sodium	Hypotonic	1/2 NS 0.45% NS
Chloride (half normal saline)		
0.9% sodium chloride (normal saline)	Isotonic	NS/0.9% NS
3%—5% sodium chloride	Hypertonic	3%—5% NS 3%—5% NaCl
Glucose (=dextrose)in saline solution		
Glucose 5% in 0.9% sodium chloride	Hypertonic	G5W&NS (D5NS)
Glucose 5% in 0.45% sodium chloride	Hypertonic	G5W&1/2NS (D51/2NS)
Multiple electrolyte solutions		
Compound sodium lactate	Isotonic	Hartmann's
Compound sodium lactate and glucose 5%	Hypertonic	Hartmann's & G5W

6-2 Peripheral Intravenous Infusion 讲解视频

Process

[Infusion Site]

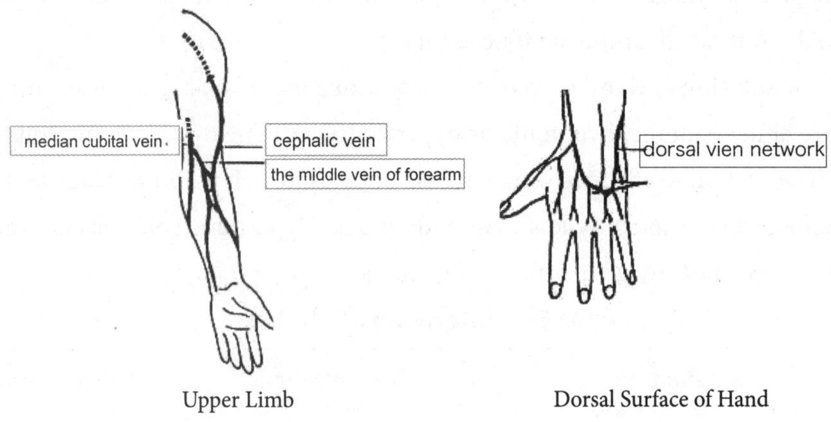

Upper Limb

Dorsal Surface of Hand

[Assessment]

Physical condition: Analyze the patient's fluid imbalance and the cardiopulmonary function, to provide the basis for safe infusion.

Selection of the puncture: Determine the puncture according to the patient's condition, infusion volume, type of solution and the patient's age, generally choose limbs superficial vein.

Psychosocial status: Assess the patient's understanding of intravenous infusion related knowledge and the patient's mental state, to provide basis for health education.

Understanding of treatment and preparation: Make sure the patient understand the purpose of IV, and empty defecate and urinate.Make sure the recumbent position is comfortable.

[Preparation]

Nurse preparation: The nurse dresses neatly, washes hands, and wears a mask.

Supply preparation: Injection plate (skin disinfectant, sterile swabs, disinfection tourniquet, garbage box), sterile syringes, infusion cards, sterile patches, disposable venous infusion, solution and drugs.

Environment preparation: Prepare environment according to the principle of sterile practice.

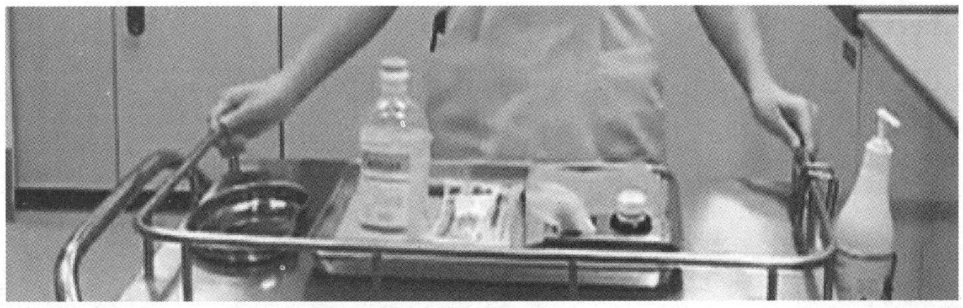

Supplies

6-3 Peripheral Intravenous Infusion 操作视频

Procedure

Step1: Check the doctor's order.

▫ The order is ready for infusion label on the bag, which indicate the bed number, name, types, dosage, and concentration (or write directly on the bag tag). Check the name of the liquid, concentration, clarity, presence of particles, suspension, etc.

Step 2: Configure solution correctly.

▫ Check again: for instance, sterile syringes, putting the drugs into the solution correctly, drugs blending in the infusion bottle. Check the quality of the solution and the signature, and indicate the time of the configuration solution (or provided directly by the configuration center).

Step 3: Insert into the bag.

▫ Disinfect infusion bag mouth again. Check the validity of infusion and the presence of air leakage. Then insert into the bag.

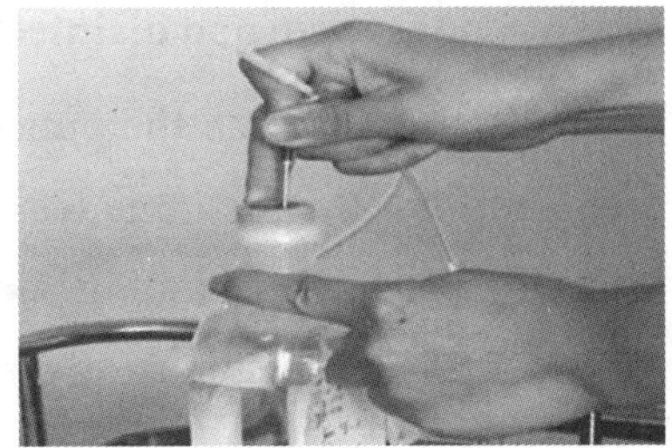

Insert into the Bag

Step 4: Check and explain.

- Check the IV information according to doctor's order again, and push items to the patient's bed. Explain the purpose of IV and duration, assist the patient to comfortable lying position, and then select the puncture site.

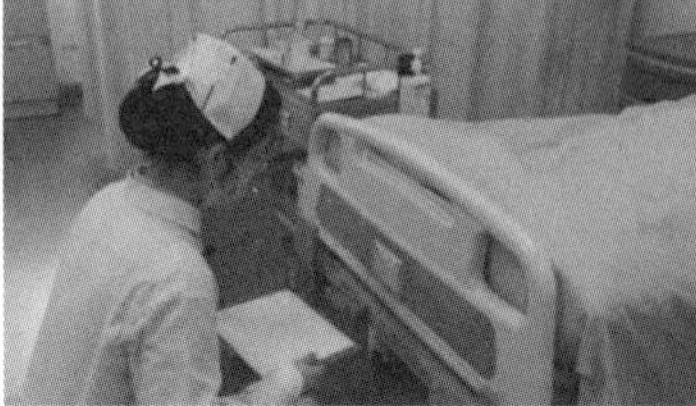

Check the Card at the End of Bed

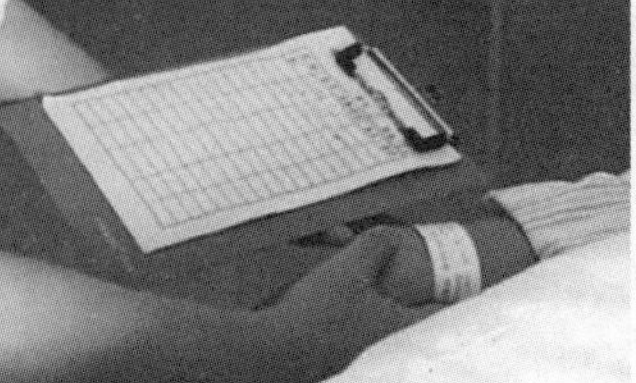

Check the Wrist Band

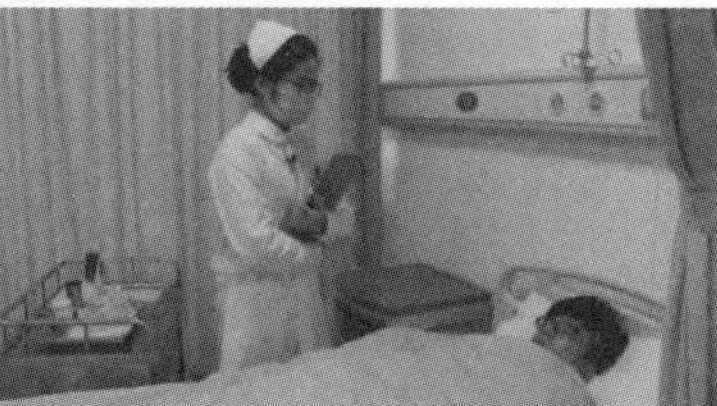

Explain

Step 5: Exhaust the air for the first time.

- Invert the microdrip and open the switch. When the liquid level is within 1/2 to 2/3 of microdrip, diverse the microdrip, slow down to make liquid outlet, and then close the regulator.

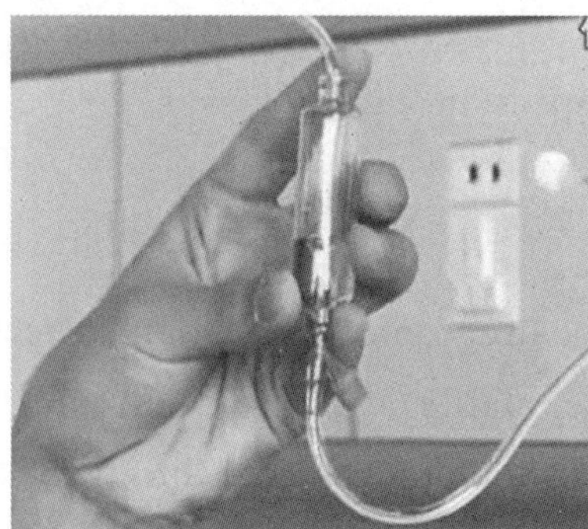

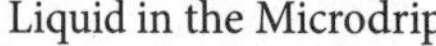

Liquid in the Microdrip

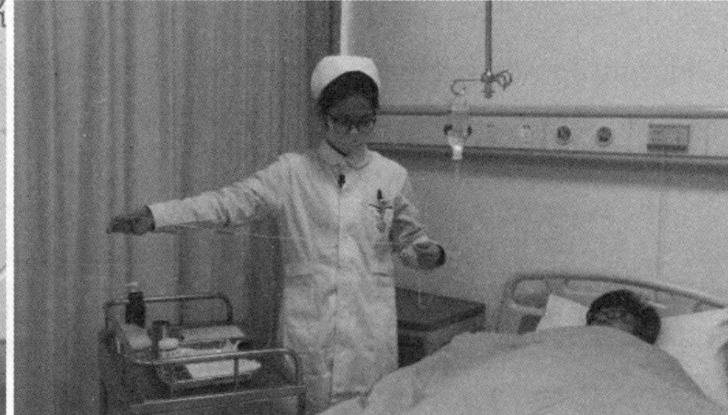

Check the Bubbles in the Tube

Step 6: Choose vein and disinfect.

- The distance between the puncture site and tourniquet is 6 cm. Sterilize the skin of the puncture for the first time (centered on the puncture site, more than 5 cm in diameter), then do patches preparation and sterilize the skin for the second time (the size is the same as the first time; disinfection direction is contrary to the first time).

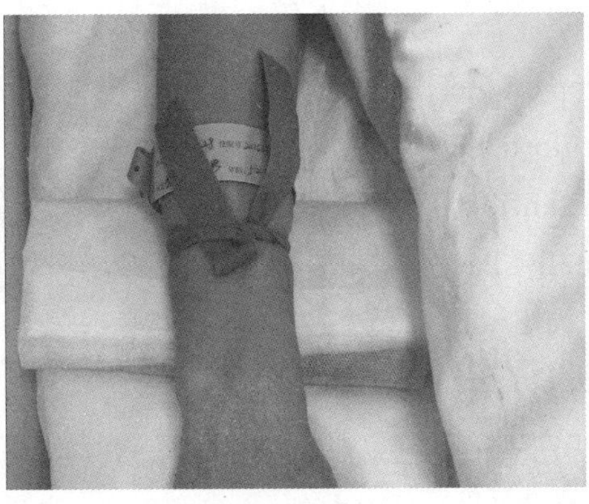

Tie the Tourniquet

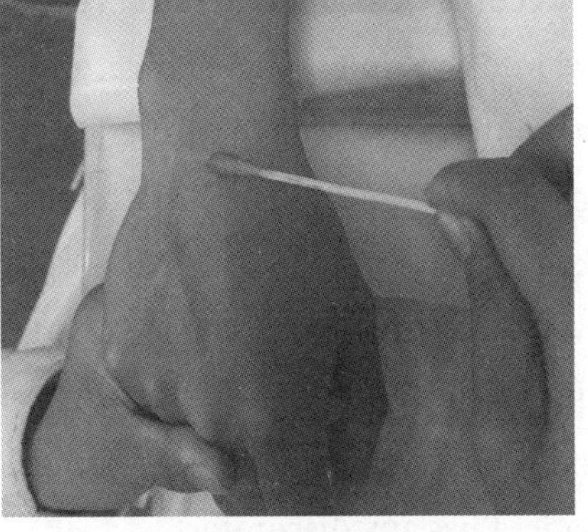

Sterile the Skin (twice)

Step 7: Exhaust the air for the second time, puncture and fix.

- Exhaust the air in the tube for the second time, then tighten skin, and insert the needle at 30—40 angle. Then insert the needle paralleled when you see the blood return. Loosen tourniquet, relax the patient's fist, and open the regulator. Then fix needle with patches, and put the patient's arm at the right place.

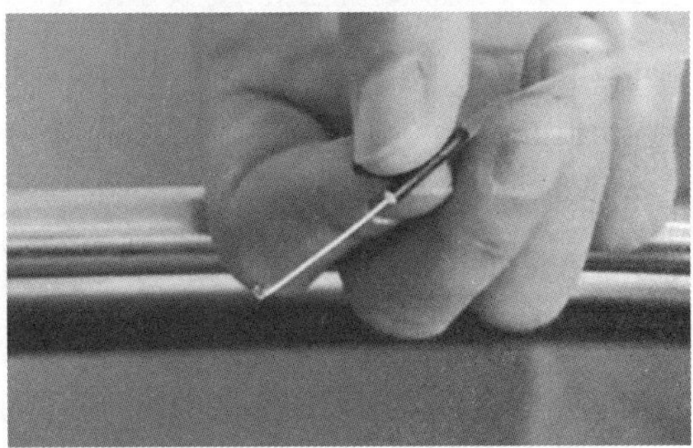

Exhaust the Air for the Second Time

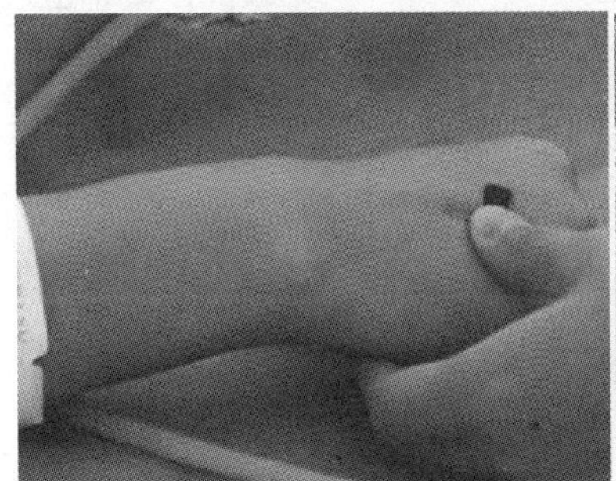

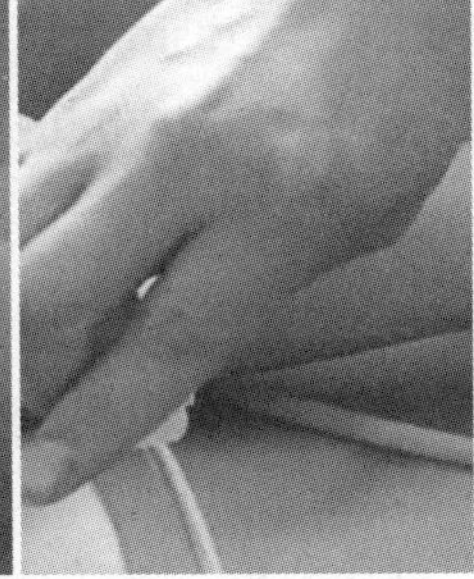

Loosen Tourniquet and Open Regulator

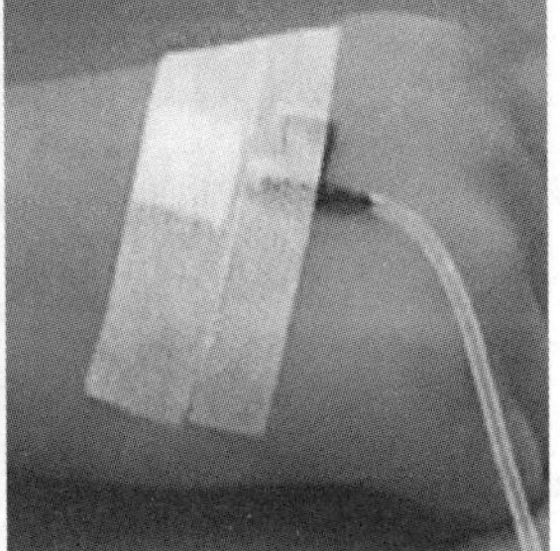

Fix Needle

Step 8: Adjust the drop.

- Adjust the drop according to the illness, age, and drug.

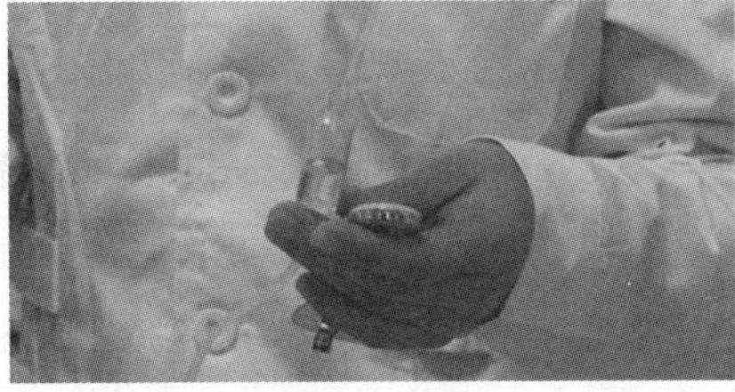

Adjust the Drop

Step 9: Record, clear up, and observe.

□ Record infusion time, drug, dosage, and drop on the IV infusion card. Assist the patient to comfortable lying position, and tell the matters of attention, for exaple, cannot adjust the drop optionally. Pay attention to infusion site, and put the call bell beside the patient before you leaving ward. During infusion, observe the patient's reaction, and ask if the patient has any discomfort.

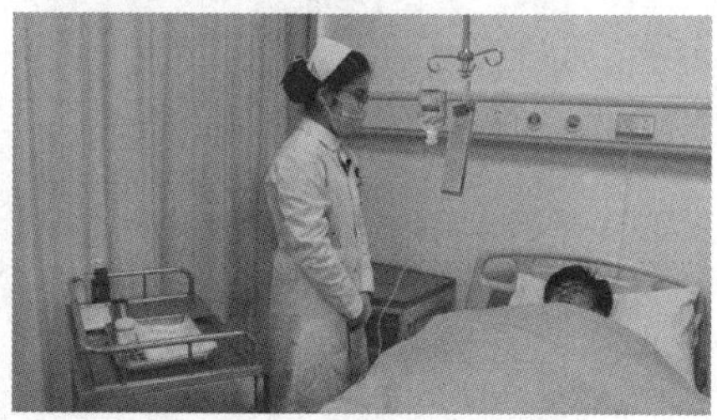

Warning

Words and Phrases

peripheral	外围的；次要的	lactate	乳酸盐
intravenous	静脉内的	median cubital vein	肘正中静脉
infusion	灌输；浸泡；注入物；激励	cephalic vein	头静脉
peripheral intravenous infusion	外周静脉输液	the middle vein of forearm	贵要静脉
electrolyte	电解液；电解质；电解	puncture	刺穿；被刺穿
acid-base balances	酸碱平衡	injection	注射
isotonic	等张的；等压的	disinfectant	消毒剂
hypotonic	低渗的；张力减退的	sterile swab	消毒棉签
hypertonic	高渗的；张力亢进的	disinfection	消毒；杀菌
osmolality	渗透度；溶质度；同渗重摩	tourniquet	止血带
saline	盐的；含盐分的	syringe	注射器
glucose	葡萄糖	patches	皮肤贴片；敷贴
sodium chloride	氯化钠；食盐	configured	配置的
		sterilize	消毒

Learning Activities

Part I Choose the best answer for each question.

1. A 30-year-old woman is admitted to the hospital with dry mucous membranes and decreased skin turgor. The woman's vital signs are BP 120/70 mmHg, temperature 101 °F (38.3 °C), pulse 88 times/min, respirations 14 times/min. Laboratory tests indicate the serum sodium is 150 mEq/L and the Hct is 48%. Which of the following IV fluids would the nurse

expect the physician to order? _______

A. D5NS.

B. 0.45% NaCl.

C. 0.9% NaCl.

D. Lactated Ringer's.

2. A patient is in the process of transfusion, cough, cough pink foam sputum, shortness of breath, sweating. Which of the following conditions may the patient appear? _______.

A. High fever

B. An allergic reaction

C.The heart overload

D. Air embolism

3. After abdominal surgery, a patient is admitted from the recovery room with intravenous fluid infusing at 100 cc/h. One hour later, the nurse finds the clamp wide open and notes that the patient has received 850 cc. Which of the following would be most concerned by the nurse? _______

A. A CVP reading of 12 and bradycardia.

B. Tachycardia and hypotension.

C. Dyspnea and oliguria.

D. Rales and tachycardia.

4. Before administering calcium gluconate 10% 500 mg IV st, it is most important for the nurse to assess the _______

A. stability of the respiratory system.

B. adequacy of urine output.

C. patency of the vein.

D. availability of magnesium sulfate injection.

5. A female patient is diagnosed with human papillomavirus (HPV). Which of the following patient's statements if made to the nurse will it illustrate an understanding of the possible sequelae of this illness? _______

A. "I will need to take antibiotics for at least a week."

B. "I will use only prescribed douches to avoid a recurrence."

C. "I will return for a Pap smear in six months."

D. "I will avoid using tampons for eight weeks."

6. A patient is being treated for hypovolemia. Which of the following observations should the nurse identify as the desired response to fluid replacement? _______

A. Urine output 160 cc/8 h.

B. Hgb 11 g, Hct 33%.

C. Arterial pH 7.34.

D. CVP reading of 8 cm of water pressure.

7. A patient in labor is receiving magnesium sulfate IV. Which assessment is most important to give during report to the nurse on the next shift? _______

A. Respiratory rate changed from 13 times/min to 15 times/min.

B. Increase in anxiety and hyperactivity.

C. Presence of nausea and refusal to take clear liquids.

D. Urine output decreased from 60 cc/h to 40 cc/h.

8. The nurse is caring for a patient with second-and third-degree burns. The patient is receiving morphine sulfate 15 mg IV. The nurse notes a decrease in bowel sounds and slight abdominal distention. Which of the following actions, taken by the nurse is the best? _______

A. Recommend that the morphine dose be decreased.

B. Withhold the pain medication.

C. Administer the medication by another route.

D. Explore alternative pain management techniques.

9. The nurse is caring for a patient receiving amphotericin B (Fungizone) 1 mg in 250 cc of 5% dextrose in water IV over a 2-hour period. Which of the following should be most concerned by the nurse? _______

A. BUN 7.2 mg/dL, creatinine 0.5 mg/dL.

B. BP 90/60 mmHg, complaints of fever and chills.

C. Complaints of burning on urination, thirst, and dizziness.

D. AST (SGOT) 12 u/l, ALT (SGPT) 14 u/l, total bilirubin 0.2 mg/dL.

10. A patient is scheduled for a cardiac catheterization at 8 AM. The patient's laboratory work was completed five days ago. The results were: K^+ 3.0 mEq/L, Na^+ 148 mEq/L, glucose 178 mg/dL. He complains of muscle weakness and cramps. Which of the following nursing actions is best? _______

A. Administer the spironolactone (Aldactone).

B. Encourage eating bananas for breakfast.

C. Obtain stat K^+ level.

D. Call for twelve-lead EKG.

11. At 11 am a patient returned to the nursing unit from the post anesthesia care unit (PACU) following a hemorrhoidectomy. At noon the patient complains of pain. The physician has ordered meperidine (Demerol) 50 mg IV q 3–4 hrs. The chart indicates that the patient was given Demerol 50 mg IV at 9:15 am. The nurse should _______

A. ask the physician if the dosage of Demerol can be increased.

B. give the patient Demerol 25 mg IV now.

C. have the patient wait until 1 PM before giving the Demerol.

D. give the patient Demerol 50 mg IV now.

12. A patient develops orthopnea, dyspnea, and basilar crackles. Which of the following nursing actions would be most appropriate for this patient? _______

A. Elevate the legs to promote venous return.

B. Decrease the IV fluids and notify the physician.

C. Orient the client to time, place, and situation.

D. Prevent complications of immobility.

Part II Case study.

Case Scenario

A 45-year-old female patient, was infusion because of flu. Five minutes after the infusion started, she found the infusion site swelling and got a pain.

Task: As her primary nurse, how to deal with this problem?

（郭玲玲　邬维娜）

Scenario Four
Postoperative Nursing

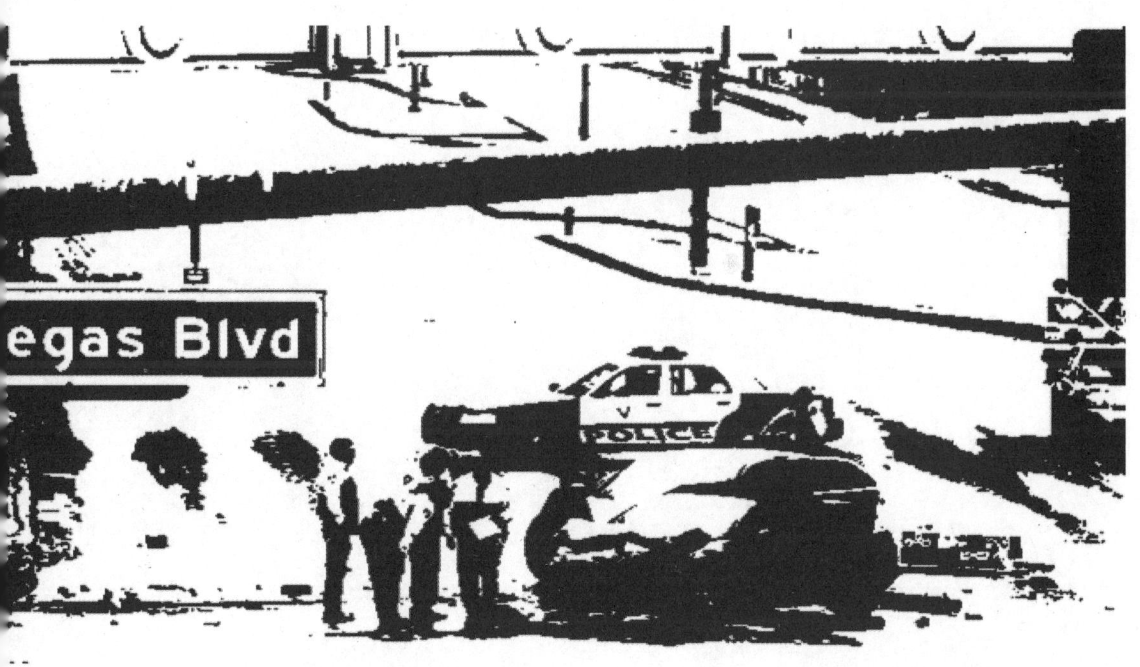

TASK 7

Replacing the Drainage

Learning Outcomes

This task will provide students with opportunities to:

- Identify the principles of postoperative management.
- Replace the drainage bag correctly.
- Cooperate with other health professionals effectively.
- Complete relative nursing documents appropriately.

Scenario

David was walking across the road after shopping for groceries when the accident happened. It occurred so suddenly that he was unable to step aside. He was heavily crashed by Mary's car and bounced five meters off. He was sent to the hospital rapidly. MRI showed he got a hepatic rupture. He had an emergency surgery immediately to save his life.

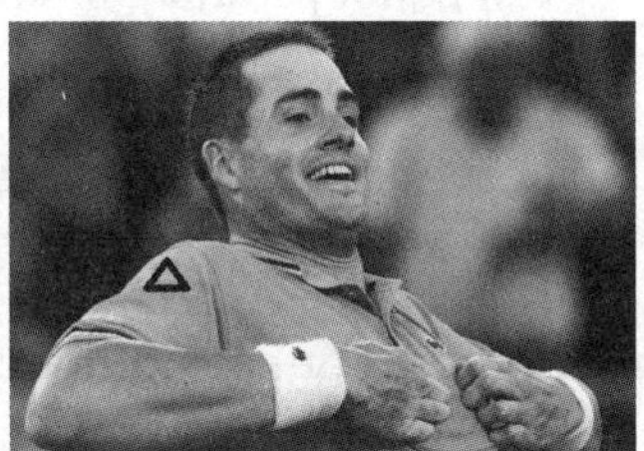

7-1 Postoperative Nursing PPT

Background

Postoperative nursing is the nursing care during the period from the patient's transfer to the recovery room or to the surgical ward. According to the patient's condition, determine the nursing problems and take effective postoperative cares. In addition, nursing measures should be implemented as soon as the patient's condition changes, in order to reduce the patient's pain and discomfort, prevent complications, as well as promote the patient's recovery.

Principles of Postoperative Management

Optimal postoperative care requires:

- Clinical assessment and monitoring.
- Respiratory management.
- Cardiovascular management.
- Fluid, electrolyte, and renal management.
- Sepsis management.
- Nutrition support.

Post-anaesthetic Recovery

Anaesthetic and surgical staff should record the following items in the patient's case notes:

- The complications related to anaesthetic, surgical or intraoperation.
- Specific postoperative instruction concerning possible problems.
- Specific treatment or prophylaxis required.

Respiratory Management

Patients in whom there is a suspicion of postoperative pulmonary complications should have an arterial blood gas analysis, a sputum culture and ECG.

Chest X-ray should be performed on suspicion of major collapse, effusion, pneumothorax or haemothorax.

Other investigations should be used only if there are specific indications.

Oxygen should be given to patients with hypoxaemia using a device that is best tolerated to achieve the necessary SpO_2.

In normally hydrated patients humidification is unnecessary.

Failure to maintain an SpO_2 >90% or PaO_2 >8.0 kPa is an indication to consider assisted ventilation.

Patients with developing respiratory failure should be referred to a critical care specialist to be assessed for possible assisted ventilation. The referral should be timely because hypoxia or hypercapnia may lead rapidly to cardio respiratory arrest.

Cardiovascular Management

Postoperative blood pressure should always be reviewed with reference to the preoperative and intraoperative assessments

Further assessment is required for patients with:

- Heart rate < 50 or > 100 bpm.
- Blood pressure <100 mmHg systolic.

Patients on regular antihypertensive medication should normally be maintained on this medication perioperatively. If the patient become hypotensive then it may be appropriate to discontinue some drugs.

Beta blockers and IV nitrates may be used safely and effectively in postoperative hypertension.

Beta blockers should be continued perioperatively in patients previously taking these drugs for coronary disease, congestive heart failure, hypertension or arrhythmias.

Be aware of clinical factors which increase risk to the patient and how these interact with the risks imposed by the surgical procedure.

Seek expert help early in the management of serious or potentially serious arrhythmias. Reconsider the level of care.

Concern the underlying causes of any supraventricular arrhythmias,eg hypoxia, hypovolemia, electrolyte abnormality, sepsis or drug toxicity.

The specialist medical advice should be sought timely once perioperative MI is diagnosed or suspected.

Maintain normothermia in the postoperative period.

Fluid, Electrolyte, and Renal Management

The fluid and electrolyte status should be monitored, and the treatment must be individualized with concerning the responses to treatment.

Volume depletion should be avoided because it can lead to poor perfusion and problems such as anastomotic breakdown, cerebral damage, renal failure and multiple organ failure. Diuretics should be reserved for fluid overload.

Hyponatremia is more commonly due to excess water than sodium deficiency assess volume status.

Hypernatremia most commonly indicates a total body deficiency of water and is an indication for prompt assessment and intervention, especially when levels exceed 155 mmol/L.

Hypokalaemia can delay postoperative recovery. Magnesium supplementation may also be required.

Metabolic acidosis is usually due to poor tissue perfusion but can also be caused by excessive administration of saline.

Sepsis Management

Hand washing with soap and water or with alcoholic cleaning agents should be performed before and after patient contact.

Early identification and appropriate treatment of sepsis improves outcome.

Urine and blood cultures should be obtained whenever there is reason to suspect systemic sepsis.

If the cause of sepsis is unknown, treat with broad spectrum antibiotics, guided by local protocols.

Results from microbiological specimens should be reviewed regularly and antibiotics changed as necessary.

A course of antimicrobial treatment should generally be limited to 5—7 days. Fungi and a typical organisms can contribute to sepsis syndrome.

Nutrition Support

Oral intake should be commenced as soon as possible after surgery.

Nutritional replacement should be discussed with a dietitian and tailored to the patient's requirements.

Enteral nutrition is the preferred method of postoperative nutritional support and should be used if possible.

Nutritional and metabolic status should be assessed regularly and the nutritional prescription modified as necessary.

Checklist for First Postoperative Assessment

Intraoperative history and postoperative instructions:

- Past medical history.
- Medications.
- Allergies.
- Intraoperative complications.
- Postoperative instructions.
- Recommended treatment & prophylaxis.

Respiratory status assessment:

- Oxygen saturation.
- Effort of breathing/use of accessory muscles.
- Respiratory rate.
- Tracheal deviation or not.
- Symmetry of respiration/expansion.
- Breath sounds.
- Percussion note.

Volume status assessment:

- Hands—warm or cool, pink or pale.
- Capillary return <2 s or not.
- Pulse rate, volume, and rhythm.
- Blood pressure.
- Conjunctival pallor.
- Jugular venous pressure.

- Urine colour and rate of production.
- Drainage from drains, wounds & NG tubes.

Mental status assessment:

- Patient conscious and normally responsive.

Record:

- Any significant symptoms, eg. chest pain, breathlessness.
- Pain and adequacy of pain control.

After specialist surgery it may be necessary to assess additional factors. The intra peritoneal drain is placed to remove excess fluid from the surgical wound site and to drain any excess fluid which can be collected in the abdominal cavity.

Intra peritoneal collections such as blood, bile, pancreatic, and intestinal fluid should be drained in order to remove contaminants, reduce the likelihood of infection, control potential anastomotic leaks, and minimize the risk of toxicity to the surrounding tissue.

How to assessment and replace the drainage bag is important in the postoperative care.

7-2 Postoperative Nursing 讲解视频

Preparation

Patient: Understand the purpose of replacement, and empty defecate and urinate. And make sure the recumbent position is comfortable.

Nurse: The nurse ought to dress neatly, have her hands washed and wear a mask.

Supply: Disposable sterile drainage bag, disposable therapeutic towel, anerdian, cotton swab, sterile gauze, latex gloves, curved plate, hemostatic forceps.

7-3 Replacing the Drainage 操作视频

Procedure

Step 1: Check.

□ Check the patient's condition and explain the purpose of replacemet.

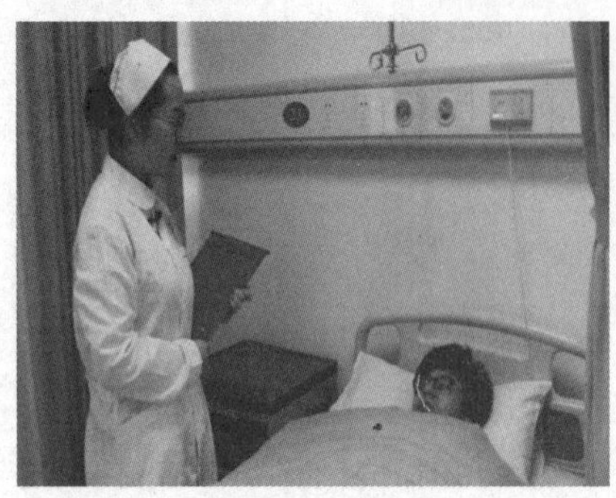

"Hello David, my name is Zounan. Can I check your wrist band? I'll change your drainage bag in order to keep it unobstructed and uninfected. I hope to get your cooperation."

Step2: Assess.

▫ Assess the wound site and the tube.

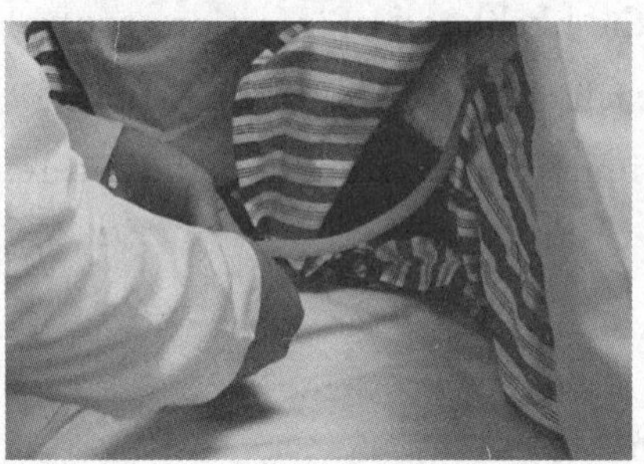

"Let me check your wound and drainage tube firstly. Please wait for a minute. I am going to get things ready and will be back immediately."

Step 3: Preparation.

▫ Take what you have prepared to the patient's room.

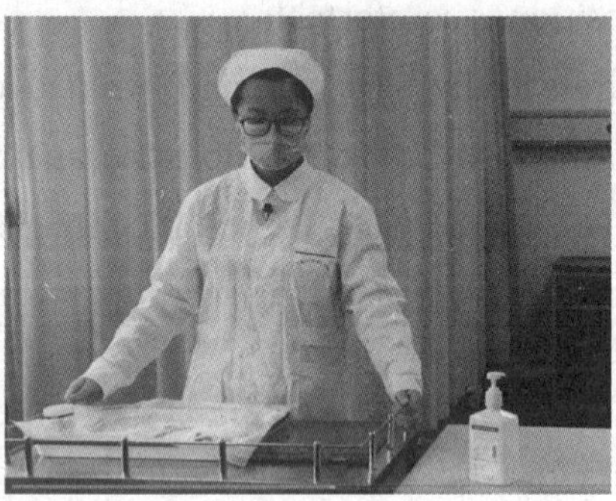

Step 4: Wash hands.

▫ Perform hand hygiene.

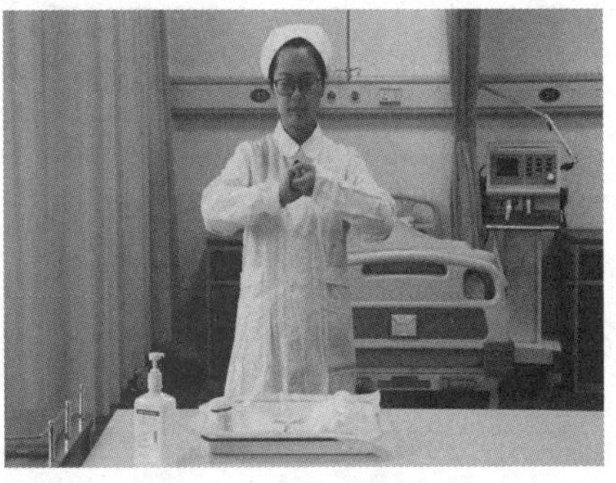

Step 5: Recheck the patient's ID.

▫ Recheck the client's ID, and assist the patient to a proper lying position.

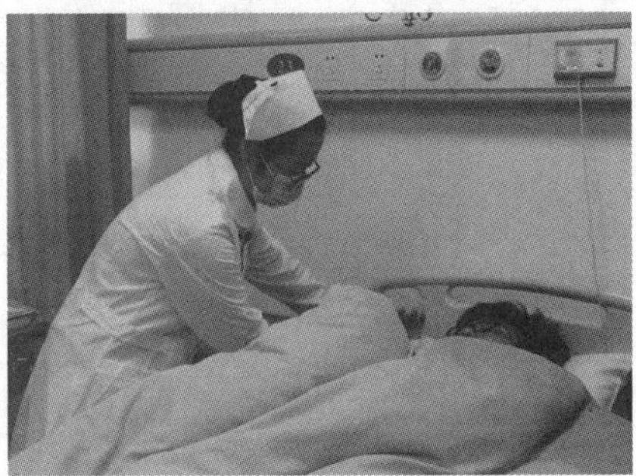

Step 6: Check the drainage bag.

▫ Open the disposable drainage bag, check whether there is any damage on the drainage bag, tighten the switch, and hang it on the bed.

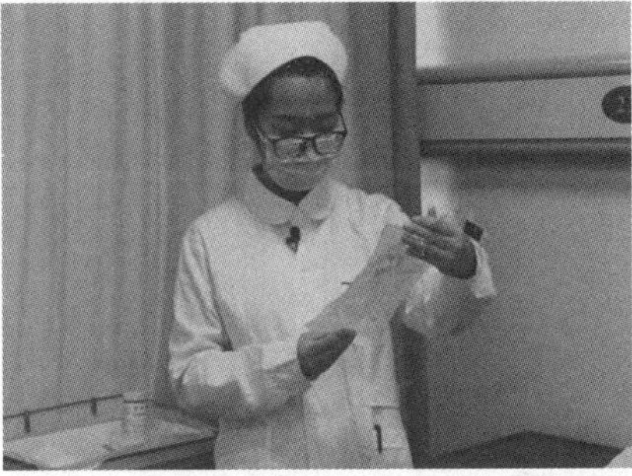

Step 7: Squeeze and clip.

▫ Clamp above the interface about 3—5 cm.

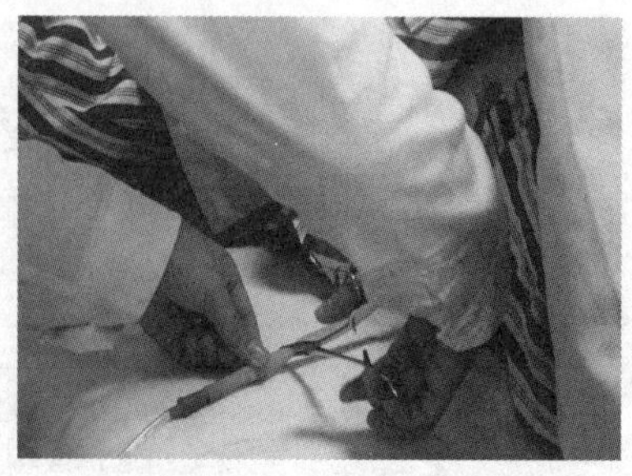

Step 8: Sterilize and replace.

- Sterilize the connection with 3 swabs, and connect the new one. Loosen the vascular clamp, then squeeze the drainage tube.

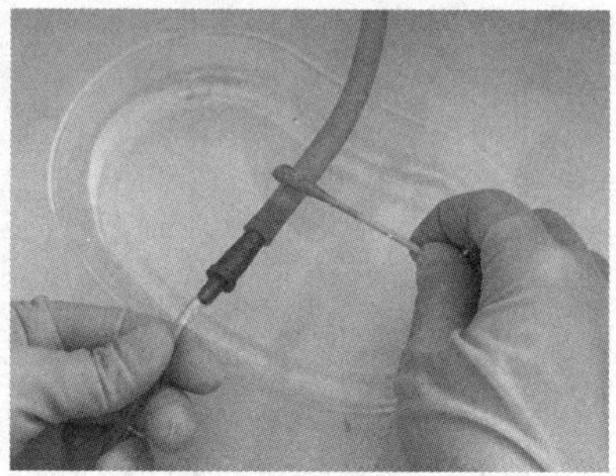

Step 9: Position the drainage bag.

- Position the drainage bag properly, and assit the patient to a comfortable lying position.

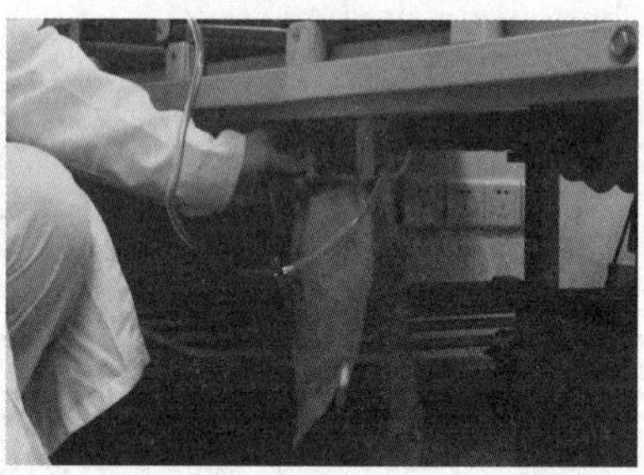

Words and Phrases

sepsis	败血症	intraperitoneal	腹腔的
deterioration	恶化	anastomotic	吻合的
antibiotics	抗生素	drainage	引流
analgesia	止痛	disposable	一次性使用的
thrombus	血栓	gloves	手套
recumbent	半卧位		

Learning Activities

Part I Choose the best answer for each question.

1. The nurse is caring for a patient who is postoperative following a pelvic exenteration and the physician changes the patient's diet from NPO status to clear liquids. Which priority assessment should the nurse make before administering the diet? ______.

A. Bowel sounds

B. Ability to ambulate

C. Incision appearance

D. Urine specific gravity

2. The nurse is caring for a patient following a mastectomy. Which assessment finding indicates that the client is experiencing a complication related to the surgery? ______.

A. Pain at the incisional site

B. Arm edema on the operative side

C. Sanguineous drainage in the Jackson-Pratt drain

D. Complaints of decreased sensation near the operative site

3. A gastrectomy is performed on a patient with gastric cancer. In the immediate postoperative period, the nurse notes bloody drainage from the nasogastric tube. Which of the following is the appropriate nursing intervention? ______.

A. Notify the physician

B. Measure abdominal girth

C. Irrigate the nasogastric tube

D. Continue to monitor the drainage

4. The nurse is assessing the perineal wound in a patient who has returned from the operating room following an abdominal perineal resection and notes serosanguineous drainage from the wound. Which nursing intervention is appropriate? ______.

A. Notify the physician

B. Clamp the Penrose drain

C. Change the dressing as prescribed

D. Remove and replace the perineal packing

5. The nurse is assessing the colostomy of a patient who has had an abdominal perineal resection for a bowel tumor. Which of the following assessment findings indicates that the colostomy is beginning to function? ______.

A. Absent bowel sounds

B. The passage of flatus

C. The patient's ability to tolerate food

D. Bloody drainage from the colostomy

6. The nurse is caring for a patient following a radical neck dissection and creation of a tracheostomy performed for laryngeal cancer and is providing discharge instructions to the patient. Which statement made by the patient indicates a need for further instructions? ___

A. "I will protect the stoma from water."

B. "I need to keep powders and sprays away from the stoma site."

C. "I need to use an air conditioner to provide cool air to assist in breathing."

D. "I need to apply a thin layer of petrolatum to the skin around the stoma to prevent cracking."

7. The nurse is caring for a patient with cancer of the prostate following a prostatectomy. The nurse provides discharge instructions to the patient and tells the patient to ______.

A. avoid driving the car for 1 week

B. restrict fluid intake to prevent incontinence

C. avoid lifting objects heavier than 20 Ib for at least 6 weeks

D. notify the physician if small blood clots are noticed during urination

8. The nurse is assessing the stoma of a patient following a ureterostomy. Which of the following should the nurse expect to note? ______.

A. A dry stoma

B. A pale stoma

C. A dark-colored stoma

D. A red and moist stoma

9. The nurse is caring for a patient following a mastectomy. Which nursing intervention would assist in preventing lymphedema of the affected arm? ______.

A. Placing cool compresses on the affected arm

B. Elevating the affected arm on a pillow above heart level

C. Avoiding arm exercises in the immediate postoperative period

D. Maintaining an intravenous site below the antecubital area on the affected side

10. The patient has just had surgery to create an ileostomy. The nurse assesses the patient in the immediate postoperative period. Which is the most frequent complication of this type of surgery? ______.

A. Folate deficiency

B. Malabsorption of fat

C. Intestinal obstruction

D. Fluid and electrolyte imbalance

Part II Case study.

Case Scenario

A 59-year-old woman with a history of diabetes and hypertension underwent a total thyroidectomy with the final pathology revealing a 3.5 cm left papillary carcinoma 24 hours ago. The nurse understands that the patient is at risk for hypocalcemia.

Task: What the nurse should do to prevent this complication?

（葛　炜　陈巍阳）

Scenario Five

Medical Nursing

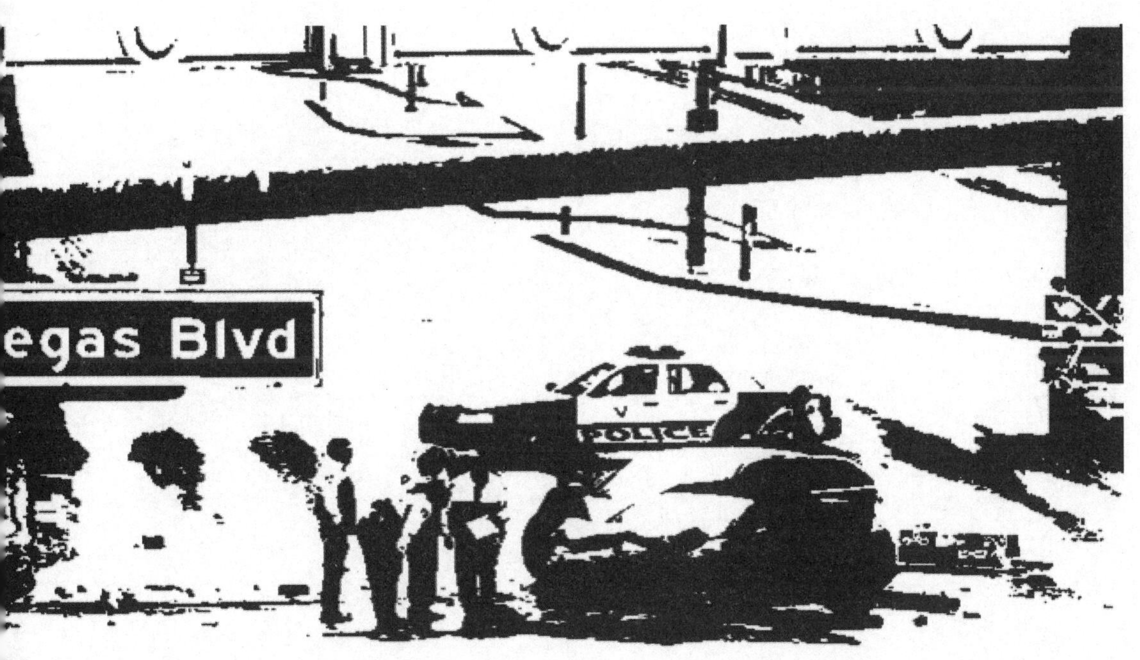

TASK 8

Chronic Obstructive Pulmonary Disease (COPD)

Learning Outcomes

This task will provide students with opportunities to:

- Describe signs and symptoms of COPD.
- Identify the risk factors of COPD.
- Understand the prevention of COPD.
- Restate the goals and techniques of pulmonary rehabilitation.
- Discuss acute exacerbations of COPD and the treatment.
- Discuss care for the patients with airflow obstruction.

Scenario

Jack, a 65-year-old man, was diagnosed with COPD 5 years ago. He was suffering from worsening dyspnea, cough, and increasing purulent sputum production over the past 3 days. On examination, BP is 130/84 mmHg, pulse 102 times/min, respiratory rate 18 times/min, and temperature 37.8 °C. Auscultation of the chest reveals widespread expiratory wheeze and inspiratory coarse crackles in the left lung base. No cyanosis is present.

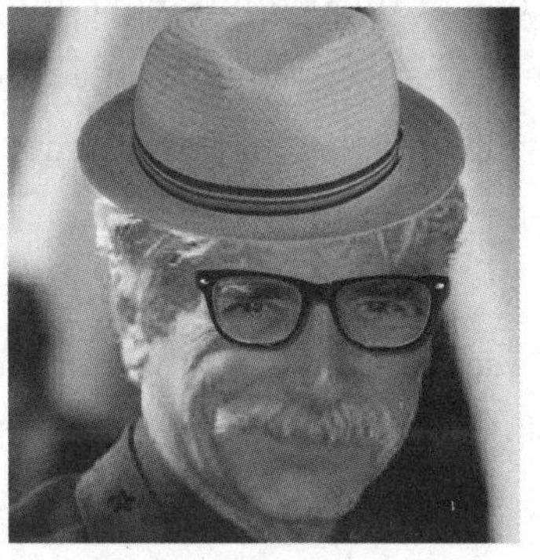

8-1 COPD PPT

Background

Chronic obstructive pulmonary disease (COPD) is a type of obstructive lung disease characterized by chronically poor airflow. It typically worsens over time. The main symptoms include shortness of breath, cough, and sputum production. Most people with chronic bronchitis have COPD.

Tobacco smoking is the most common cause of COPD, with a number of other factors such as air pollution and genetics playing a smaller role. In the developing world, one of the common sources of air pollution is from poorly vented cooking and heating fires. Long-term exposure to these irritants causes an inflammatory response in the lungs resulting in narrowing of the small airways and breakdown of lung tissue known as emphysema. The diagnosis is based on poor airflow as measured by lung function tests. In contrast to asthma, the airflow reduction does not improve significantly with the administration of medication.

COPD can be prevented by reducing exposure to the known causes. This includes efforts to decrease rates of smoking and to improve indoor and outdoor air quality. COPD treatments include quitting smoking, vaccinations, rehabilitation, and often inhaled bronchodilators and steroids. Some people may benefit from long-term oxygen therapy or nursing interventions or lung transplantation. In those who have periods of acute worsening, increased use of medications and hospitalization may be needed.

Symptoms

The most common symptoms of COPD are sputum production, shortness of breath, and a productive cough. These symptoms are present for a prolonged period of time and typically worsen over time. It is unclear if different types of COPD exist. While previously divided into emphysema and chronic bronchitis, emphysema is only a description of lung changes rather than a disease itself, and chronic bronchitis is simply a descriptor of symptoms that may or may not occur with COPD.

- **Cough**

A chronic cough is usually the first symptom to occur. When it exists for more than three months a year for more than two years, in combination with sputum production and without another explanation, there is by definition chronic bronchitis. This condition can occur before COPD fully develops. The amount of sputum produced can change over hours to days. In some cases the cough may not be present or only occurs occasionally and may not be productive. Some people with COPD attribute the symptoms to a "smoker's cough." Sputum may be swallowed or spat out, depending often on social and cultural factors. Vigorous coughing may lead to rib fractures or a brief loss of consciousness. Those with COPD often have a history of "common colds" that last a long time.

- **Shortness of breath**

Shortness of breath is the symptom that most people complained. It is commonly described as "my breathing requires effort," "I feel out of breath," or "I can't get enough air in." Different terms, however, may be used in different cultures. Typically the shortness of breath is worse on exertion of a prolonged duration and worsens over time. In the advanced stages it occurs during rest and may be always present. It is a source of both anxiety and a poor quality of life in those with COPD. Many people with more advanced COPD breathe through pursed lips and this action can improve shortness of breath in some way.

- **Other features**

In COPD, it may take longer to breathe out than to breathe in. Chest tightness may occur, but it is not common and may be caused by another problem. Those with obstructed airflow may have wheezing or decreased sounds with air entry on examination of the chest with a stethoscope. A barrel chest is a characteristic sign of COPD, but is relatively uncommon. Tripod positioning may occur as the disease worsens.

- **Exacerbation**

An acute exacerbation of COPD is defined as increased shortness of breath, increased sputum production, a change in the color of the sputum from clear to green or yellow, or an increase in cough in someone with COPD. This may present with signs of increased work of breathing such as fast breathing, a fast heart rate, sweating, active use of muscles in the neck, a bluish tinge to the skin, and confusion or combative behavior in very severe exacerbations. Crackles may also be heard over the lungs on examination with a stethoscope.

Pathophysiology

COPD is a type of obstructive lung disease in which chronic incompletely reversible poor airflow (airflow limitation) and inability to breath out fully (air trapping) exist. The poor airflow is the result of breakdown of lung tissue (known as emphysema) and small airways disease known as obstructive bronchiolitis. The relative contributions of these two factors vary between people. Severe destruction of small airways can lead to the formation of large air pockets—known as bullae—that replace lung tissue. This form of disease is called bullous emphysema.

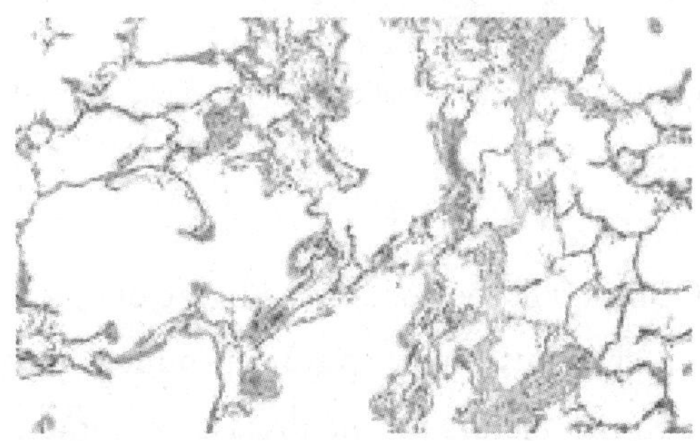

Micrograph showing emphysema (left-large empty spaces) and lung tissue with relative preservation of the alveoli (right).

Narrowing of the airways occurs due to inflammation and scarring within them. This contributes to the inability to breathe out fully. The greatest reduction in air flow occurs when breathing out, as the pressure in the chest is compressing the airways at this time.

This can result in more air from the previous breath remaining within the lungs when the next breath is started, resulting in an increase in the total volume of air in the lungs at any given time, a process called hyperinflation or air trapping. Hyperinflation from exercise is linked to shortness of breath in COPD, as it is less comfortable to breathe in when the lungs are already partly full. Some also have a degree of airway hyperresponsiveness to irritants similar to those found in asthma.

Low oxygen levels and, eventually, high carbon dioxide levels in the blood can occur from poor gas exchange due to decreased ventilation from airway obstruction, hyperinflation, and a reduced desire to breathe. During exacerbations, airway inflammation is also increased, resulting in increased hyperinflation, reduced expiratory airflow, and worsening of gas transfer. This can also lead to insufficient ventilation and, eventually, low blood oxygen levels. Low oxygen levels, if present for a prolonged period, can result in narrowing of the arteries in the lungs, while emphysema leads to breakdown of capillaries in the lungs. Both these changes result in increased blood pressure in the pulmonary arteries, which may cause corpulmonale.

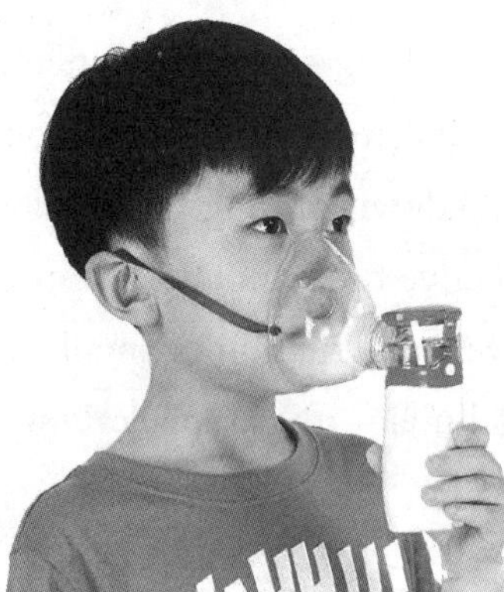

A person is blowing into a spirometer. Smaller handheld devices are available for office use.

- **Diagnosis**

The diagnosis of COPD should be considered in anyone over the age of 35 to 40 who has shortness of breath, a chronic cough, sputum production, or frequent winter colds and a history of exposure to risk factors for the disease. Spirometry is used to diagnose the disease.

- **Spirometry**

Spirometry is used to measure the severity of airflow obstruction. It is generally carried out after a bronchodilator treatment. Two main components are measured to make the diagnosis: the forced expiratory volume in one second (FEV1), which is the greatest volume of air that can be breathed out in the first second of a breath, and the forced vital capacity

(FVC), which is the greatest volume of air that can be breathed out in a single large breath. Normally, 75%—80% of the FVC comes out in the first second and a FEV1/FVC ratio of less than 70% in someone with symptoms of COPD defines a person having the disease. Based on these measurements, spirometry would lead to over-diagnosis of COPD in the elderly. The National Institute for Health and Care Excellence criteria additionally require a FEV1 of less than 80% of predicted.

- **Other tests**

A chest X-ray and complete blood count may be useful to exclude other conditions at the time of diagnosis. Characteristic signs on X-ray are over expanded lungs, a flattened diaphragm, increased retrosternal airspace, and bullae while it can help exclude other lung diseases, such as pneumonia, pulmonary edema or a pneumothorax. A high-resolution computed tomography scan of the chest may show the distribution of emphysema in lungs and can also be useful to exclude other lung diseases, complications, as well as promote the patient's recovery.

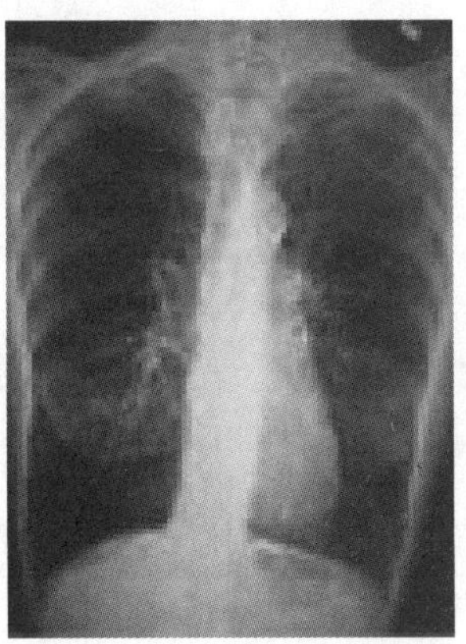

Chest X-ray demonstrates severe COPD. Note the small heart size in comparison to the lungs.

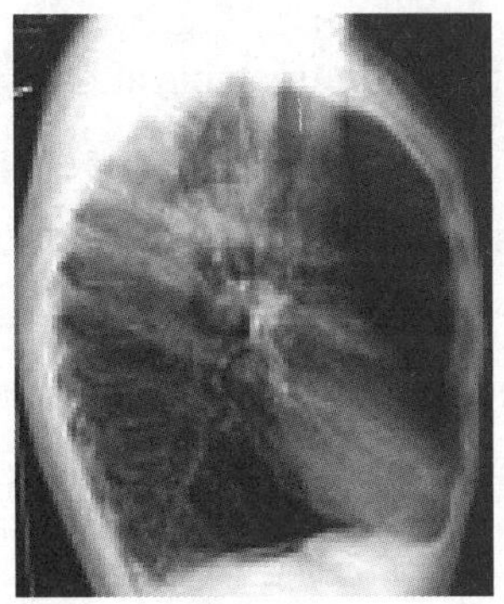

A lateral chest x-ray of a person with emphysema. Note the barrel chest and flat diaphragm.

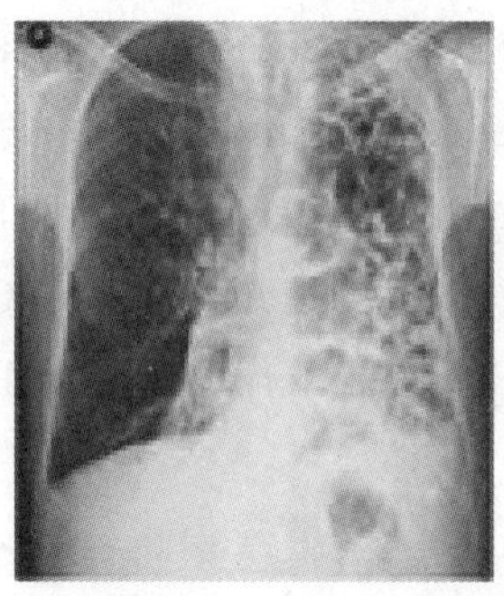

A severe case of bullous emphysema

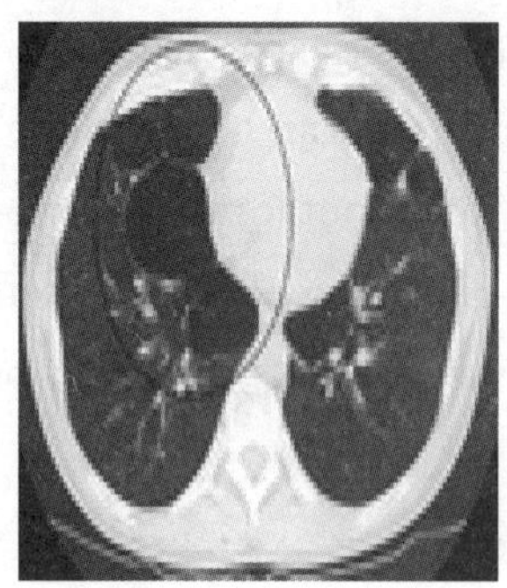

Axial CT image of the lung of a person with end-stage bullous emphysema.

8-2 COPD 讲解视频

Prevention

Most cases of COPD are potentially preventable through decreasing exposure to smoke and improving air quality. Annual influenza vaccinations in those with COPD reduce exacerbations, hospitalizations and death. Pneumococcal vaccination may also be beneficial.

- **Management**

There is no known cure for COPD, but the symptoms are treatable and its progression can be delayed. The major goals of management are to reduce risk factors, manage stable COPD, prevent and treat acute exacerbations, and manage associated illnesses. The only measures that have been shown to reduce mortality are smoking cessation and supplemental oxygen. Other recommendations include influenza vaccination once a year, pneumococcal vaccination once every 5 years, and reduction in exposure to environmental air pollution.

- **Exercise**

Pulmonary rehabilitation is a program of exercise, disease management and counseling, coordinated to benefit the individual. In those who have had a recent exacerbation, pulmonary rehabilitation appears to improve the overall quality of life and the ability to exercise, and reduce mortality. It has also been shown to improve the sense of control a person has over their disease, as well as their emotions. The exercises include providing respiratory treatments and CPT and instructing the patient in diaphragmatic or abdominal techniques and pursed-lip breathing techniques.

Being either underweight or overweight can affect the symptoms, degree of disability and prognosis of COPD. People with COPD who are underweight can improve their breathing muscle strength by increasing their calorie intake. When combined with regular exercise or a pulmonary rehabilitation program, this can lead to improvements in COPD symptoms.

- **Bronchodilators**

Inhaled bronchodilators are the primary medications used and result in a small overall benefit. There are two major types, β2 agonists and anticholinergics; both exist in long-acting and short-acting forms. They reduce shortness of breath, wheeze and exercise limitation, resulting in an improved quality of life.

- **Corticosteroids**

Corticosteroids are usually used in inhaled form but may also be used as tablets to treat and prevent acute exacerbations. While inhaled corticosteroids have not shown benefit for people with mild COPD, they decrease acute exacerbations in those with either moderate or severe disease.

- **Other medication**

Long-term antibiotics, specifically those from the macrolide class such as erythromycin, reduce the frequency of exacerbations in those who have the disease two years or more than a year.

- **Oxygen**

Supplemental oxygen is recommended in those who are with low oxygen levels at rest (a partial pressure of oxygen of less than 50—55 mm Hg or oxygen saturations of less than 88%). In this group of people it decreases the risk of heart failure and death if used 15 hours per day and may improve people's ability to exercise. In those who are with normal or mildly low oxygen levels, oxygen supplementation may improve shortness of breath. Administer a low concentration of oxygen(1 to 2 L/min) as prescribed; the stimulus to breathe is a low arterial PO_2 instead of an increased PCO_2.

- **Surgery**

For those who are with very severe disease surgery is sometimes helpful and may include lung transplantation or lung volume reduction surgery. Lung volume reduction surgery involves removing the parts of the lung most damaged by emphysema allowing the remaining, relatively good lung to expand and work better. Lung transplantation is sometimes performed for very severe COPD, particularly in younger individuals.

- **Other interventions**

Provide respiratory treatments and CPT, at the same time instruct the patient in diaphragmatic or abdominal techniques and pursed-lip breathing techniques.

Process

[Client Instruction for Incentive Spirometry]

□ Instruct the patient to assume a sitting or upright position and place the mouth tightly around the mouthpiece of the device.

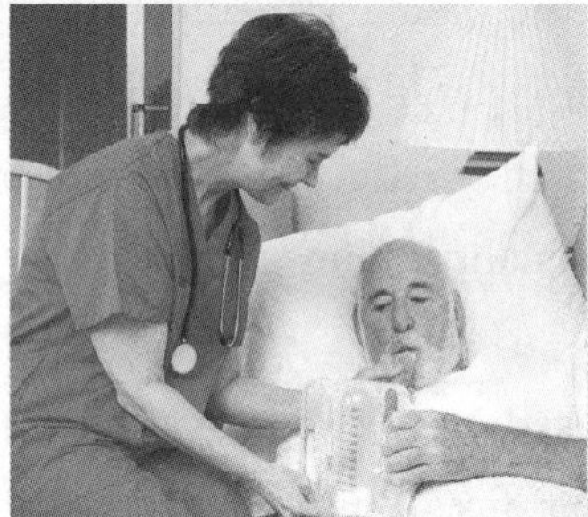

□ Instruct the patient to inhale slowly to raise and maintain the flow rate indicator between the 600 and 900 marks, at the same time, hold the breath for 5 seconds and then to exhale through pressed lips.

□ Instruct the patient to repeat this process 10 times every hour.

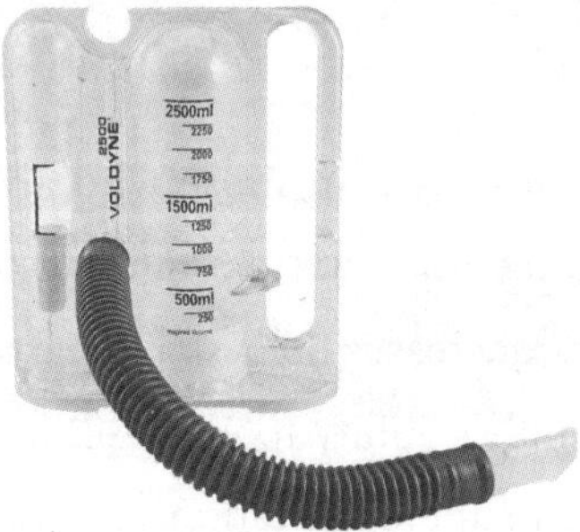

[Respiratory Treatments]

Breathing retraining: This includes exercises to decrease the use of accessory muscles of breathing to decrease fatigue and to promote CO_2 elimination. The main types of exercises include pursed-lip breathing and diaphragmatic breathing.

▫ The patient should place the hand over the abdomen while inhaling slowly through the nose; the abdomen should expand with inhalation and contract during exhalation.

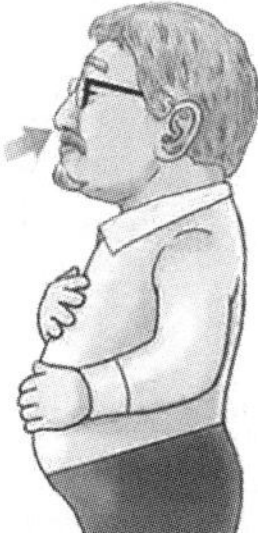

▫ The patient should exhale three times longer than inhalation by blowing through pursed lips.

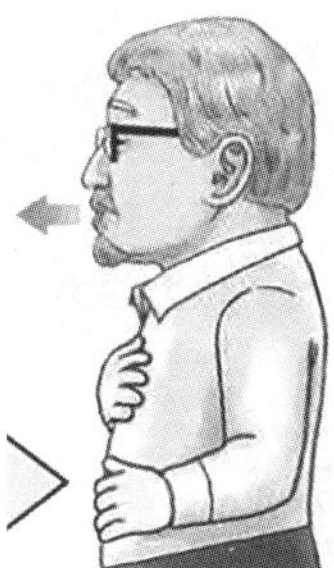

Chest physiotherapy (CPT): Percussion, vibration, and postural drainage techniques are performed over the thorax to loosen secretions in the affected area of the lungs and move them into more central airways. Perform CPT in the morning on arising, 1 hour before meals, or 2 to 3 hours after meals. If the patient is receiving a tube feeding, stop the feeding and aspirate the residual before beginning CPT, and administer the bronchodilator (if prescribed) 15 minutes before the procedure.

▫ Place a layer of material (gown or pajamas) between the hands or percussion device and the patient's skin, and position the patient for postural drainage based on assessment.
▫ Percuss the area for 1 to 2 minutes.

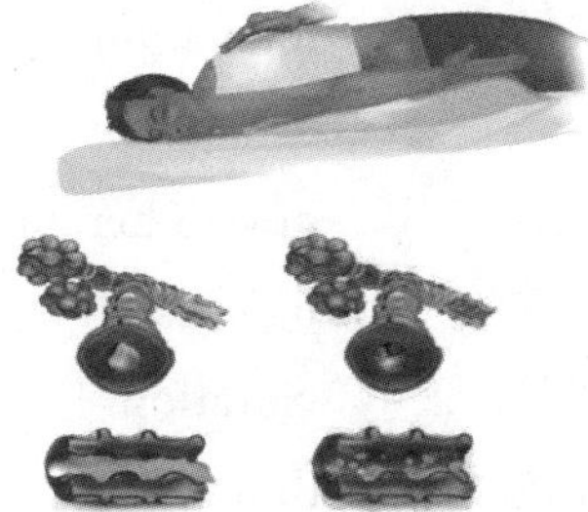

- Vibrate the same area while the patient exhales four or five deep breaths.
- Repeat in all necessary position until the patient no longer expectorates mucus.

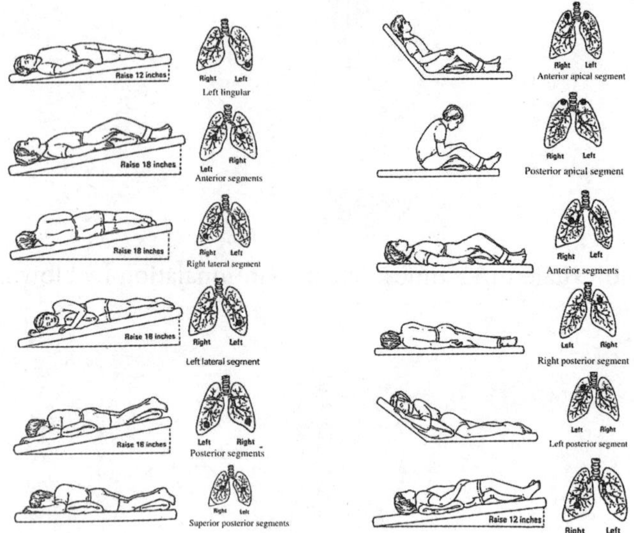

8-3 COPD 操作视频

Words and Phrases

pulmonary	肺的；肺部的
bronchitis	支气管炎
Inflammatory	发炎的；炎性的
emphysema	肺气肿
asthma	哮喘；喘息；哮喘病
vaccination	预防接种
bronchodilator	支气管扩张药
sputum	痰液
stethoscope	听诊器
exacerbation	病势加重
pathophysiology	病理生理学
alveoli	肺泡
hyperinflation	过度膨胀
capillary	毛细血管
spirometer	呼吸量测定器
diaphragm	横膈膜
pneumonia	肺炎
corticosteroid	(肾上腺)皮质激素类
pursed-lip	缩唇
inhalation	吸气
exhalation	呼气
physiotherapy	理疗
percussion	叩诊；敲打；冲击
vibration	振动；摆动
thorax	胸；胸部；胸腔

Learning Activities

Part I Choose the best answer for each question.

1. A nurse is caring for a patient hospitalized with acute exacerbation of chronic obstructive pulmonary disease. Which of the following would the nurse expect to note on assessment of this patient? _______.

A. Hypocapnia

B. A hyper inflated chest noted on the chest X-ray

C. Increased oxygen saturation with exercise

D. A widened diaphragm noted on the chest X-ray

2. An oxygen delivery system is prescribed for a patient with chronic obstructive pulmonary disease to deliver a precise oxygen concentration. Which of the following types of oxygen delivery systems would the nurse anticipate to be prescribed? _______.

A. Face tent

B. Venturi mask

C. Aerosol mask

D. Tracheostomy collar

3. A nurse instructs a patient to use the pursed-lip method of breathing and the patient asks the nurse about the purpose of this type of breathing. The nurse responds, knowing that the primary purpose of pursed-lip breathing is to _______.

A. promote oxygen intake

B. strengthen the diaphragm

C. strengthen the intercostals muscles

D. promote carbon dioxide elimination

4. A nurse is assessing a patient with chronic airflow limitation and notes that the patient has a "barrel chest." Which of the following forms of chronic airflow limitation does the nurse interpret that this client has? _______.

A. Emphysema

B. Bronchial asthma

C. Chronic obstructive bronchitis

D. Bronchial asthma and bronchitis

5. When performing an assessment on the patient with emphysema, the nurse finds that the patient has a barrel chest. The alteration in the patient's chest is due to _______.

A. collapse of distal alveoli

B. hyperinflation of the lungs

C. long-term chronic hypoxia

D. use of accessory muscles

6. The nurse notes that a patient with COPD demonstrates more dyspnea in certain positions. Which position is most likely to alleviate the patient's dyspnea? _______.

A. Lying supine with a single pillow

B. Standing or sitting upright

C. Side-lying with the head elevated

D. Lying with head slightly lowered

7. When reviewing the chart of a patient with long standing lung disease, which pulmonary function test should the nurse pay close attention to the results of? _______.

A. Residual volume

B. Total lung capacity

C. FEV1/FVC ratio

D. Functional residual capacity

8. The physician has ordered O_2 at 3 liters/min via nasal cannula. O_2 amounts greater than 3 liters/min are contraindicated in the patient with COPD because _______.

A. higher concentrations result in severe headache

B. hypercapnic drive is necessary for breathing

C. higher levels will be required later to raise the PO_2

D. hypoxic drive is needed for breathing

9. A nurse is instructing a hospitalized patient with a diagnosis of emphysema about measures that will enhance the effectiveness of breathing during dyspneic periods. Which of the following positions will the nurse instruct the patient to assume? _______.

A. Sitting up in bed

B. Side-lying in bed

C. Sitting in a recliner chair

D. Sitting on the side of the bed and leaning on an overbed table

10. A nurse is caring for a patient with emphysema. The patient is receiving oxygen. The nurse assesses the oxygen flow rate to ensure that it does not exceed _______.

A. 1 L/min

B. 2 L/min

C. 6 L/min

D. 10 L/min

Part II Case study

Case Scenario

A 69-year-old patient appears thin and cachectic. He is short of breath at rest and has dyspnea increases with the slightest exertion. His breath sounds are diminished even with deep inspiration.

Task: What is the matter with the patient?

（陈　燕　乔　乔）

TASK 9

Applying Oxygen and Suctioning

Learning Outcomes

This task will provide students with opportunities to:

- Apply the nasal cannula properly to deliver oxygen.
- Identify unexpected outcomes associated with the oxygen delivery device and the need to notify the physician if any occur.
- Take proper actions to perform respiratory suctioning.
- Identify unexpected outcomes associated with respirtory suctioning and the need to notify the physician if any occur.
- Cooperate and communicate with other health care workers effectively. Complete related nursing documents appropriately.

Scenario

Jack, a 65-year-old man, was diagnosed with COPD 5 years ago. He presents with worsening dyspnea, cough, and increasing purulent sputum production over the past 3 days. On examination, BP is 130/84 mmHg, pulse 102 times/min, respiratory rate 18 times/min, and temperature 37.8 °C. Auscultation of the chest reveals widespread expiratory wheeze and inspiratory coarse crackles in the left lung base. No cyanosis is present.

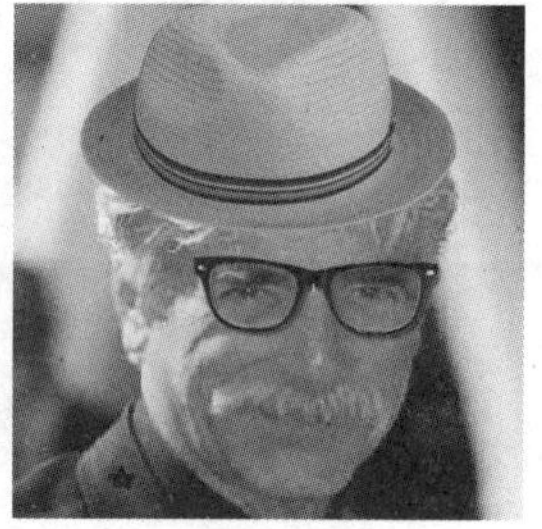

9-1 Pipeline Care PPT

Background

Gas Transport

The oxygen transport system consists of the lungs and cardiovascular system. Delivery depends on the amount of oxygen entering the lungs ventilation, blood flow to the lungs and tissues(perfusions), rate of diffusion, and oxygen-carrying capacity. The capacity of the blood to carry oxygen in the plasma lies on the amount of hemoglobin, and tendency of hemoglobin to bind with oxygen. Only a relatively small amount of required oxygen, less than 1%, is dissolved in the plasma. Most oxygen is transported by hemoglobin in the red blood cells, which serves as a carrier for oxygen and carbon dioxide. The oxygen is released to the cells as needed. Carbon dioxide is carried in several ways but is mostly converted to an acid called carbonic acid.

Regulation of Respiration

Regulation of respiration is very important to ensure sufficient oxygen intake and carbon dioxide elimination to meet the body's demands. Neural regulation including the central nervous system controls respiration rate, depth, and rhythm. Chemical regulation involves the influence of chemicals such as carbon dioxide and hydrogen ions on the rate and depth of respiration. The amount of carbon dioxide that is exhaled is important in regulating the acidity or alkalinity of the blood, based on the amount of carbonic acid that is formed. Dangerous shifts in blood pH can result from too much or too little carbon dioxide being exhaled.

9-2 Oxygen Management讲解视频

9-3 Suctioning 讲解视频

Process

[Assessment]

Physical condition: Analyze the patient's cardiopulmonary function, to provide the basis for safe suctioning and oxygen apply.

Psychosocial status: Assess patient's understanding of suctioning and oxygen applying related knowledge and the paient's mental state, to provide basis for health education.

Understanding of treatment and preparation: Make sure the patient understand the purpose of suctioning and oxygen applying, and empty defecate and urinate. Make sure the recumbent position is comfortable.

[Preparation]

Nurse: The nurse dresses neatly, washes hands, and wears a mask.

Oxygen equipment: Nasal cannula, oxygen tubing, humidifier, sterile water for humidifier, oxygen source, oxygen flow meter, oxygen in use sign.

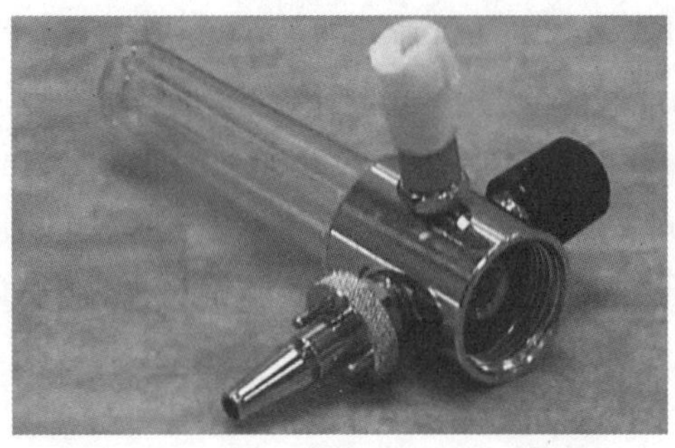
Oxygen Flowmeter

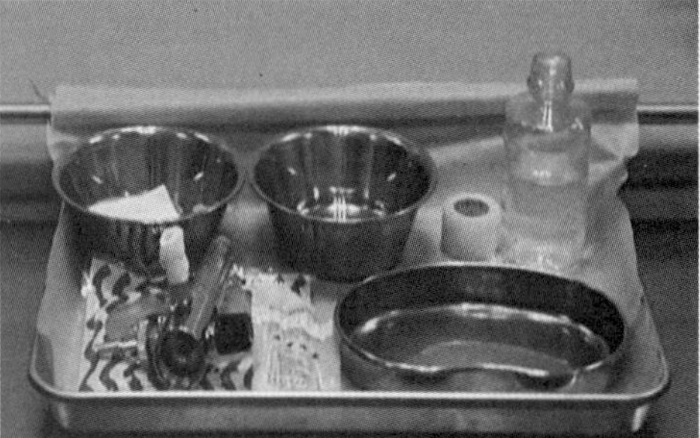
Supplies

Suctioning equipment: Appropriate-site suction catheter, two sterile gloves, sterile normal saline solution, clean towel, portable suction unit or wall suction (medical central suction system), connecting tube, mask.

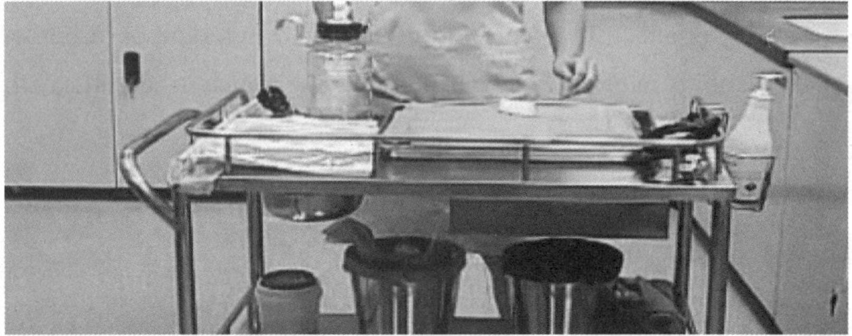
Supplies of Suctioning

Environment preparation: Prepare a safe and quiet environment according to the principle of sterile practice when practice suctioning.

9-4 Oxygen Management 操作视频

Procedure

Applying Oxygen

Step1: Inspect the patient.

- Inspect the patient for signs and symptoms associated with hypoxia and presence of airway secretions.

Step 2: Check and explain.

- Explain the procedure to the patient and family for the purpose of oxygen therapy, then wash hands.

Step 3: Oxygen.

- Connect the humidification bottle to oxygen tubing. Attach nasal cannual to the oxygen therapy device and adjust to prescribed flow rate.
- Place the nasal prongs in the nostrils, with the openings facing the patient. Adjust elastic head band or plastic slide until cannula fits snugly and comfortably.

Step 4: Check again and explain.

- Check cannula every 8 hours and check the water level. Change the humidifier as needed.
- Assess the nasal mucosa because high flow rates have a drying effect and increase mucosal irritation.
- Assess skin integrity because the oxygen tubing can irritate the skin.
- Check oxygen flow rate and doctor's order every 8 hours.
- Wash hands.
- Assess the patient for changes in respiratory rate or depth.

9-5 Suctioning 操作视频

Suctioning

Step 1: Assess the patient.

- Assess signs and symptoms of upper and lower airway obstruction requiring nasotracheal or orotracheal suctioning, including respiratory rate or rales, nasal secretions, saliva, gastric secretions or vomitus in mouth. Assess signs and symptoms associated with hypoxia and hypercapnia: apprehension, anxiety, decreased ability to concentrate, lethargy, decreased level of consciousness, increased fatigue, dizziness, behavioural changes, increased pulse rate or rate of breathing, decreased depth of breathing, elevated blood pressure, cardiac dysrhythmias, pallor, cyanosis and dyspnea.
- Assess the patient's understanding of procedure.
- Obtain doctor's order if indicated by agency policy.
- Explain the procedure to the patient . Encourage the patient to cough out secretions. Practice coughing, if possible.

- Help the patient adjust to a comfortable position.

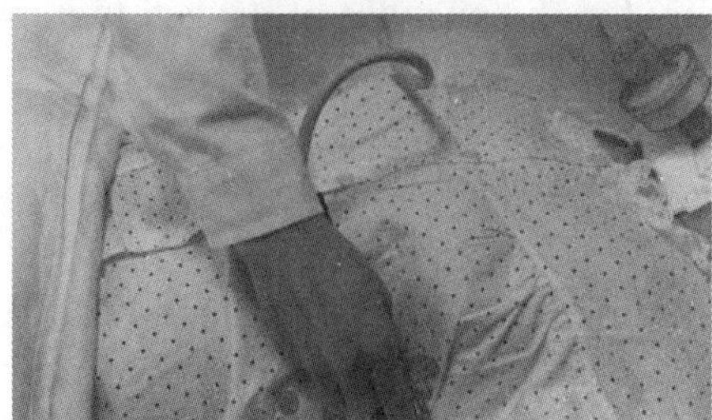
Assess

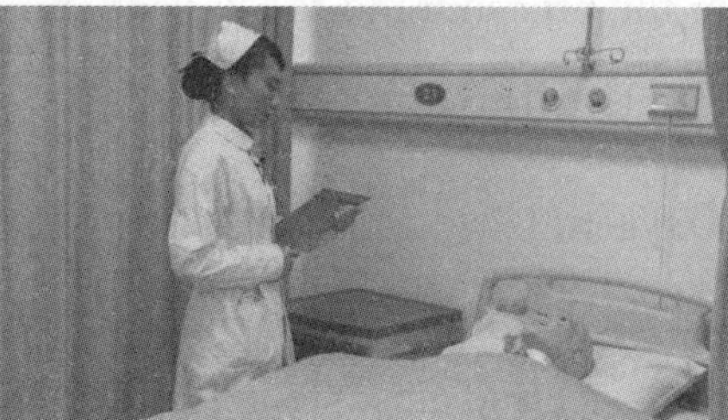
Explain

Step 2: Prepar for suctioning.

- Place towel across the patient's chest. Connect tubing to suction machine and place other end in convenient location near the patient.
- Turn suction device on and set vacuum regulator to appropriate negative pressure.
- If indicated, increase supplemental oxygen therapy to 100% or as ordered by doctor. Encourage the patient to take deep breaths.
- Prepare suction catheter: open suction catheter with use of aseptic technique.
- If sterile drape is available, place it across the patient's chest or on the over bed table. Do not allow the suction catheter to touch any non-sterile surfaces. Open sterile basin and place on beside table. Be careful not to touch inside of basin.
- Fill with about 100 ml of sterile normal saline solution or water.
- Put sterile glove on each hand.
- Pick up suction catheter with dominant hand without touching non-sterile surface. Pick up connecting tubing with non-dominant hand. Secure catheter to tubing.

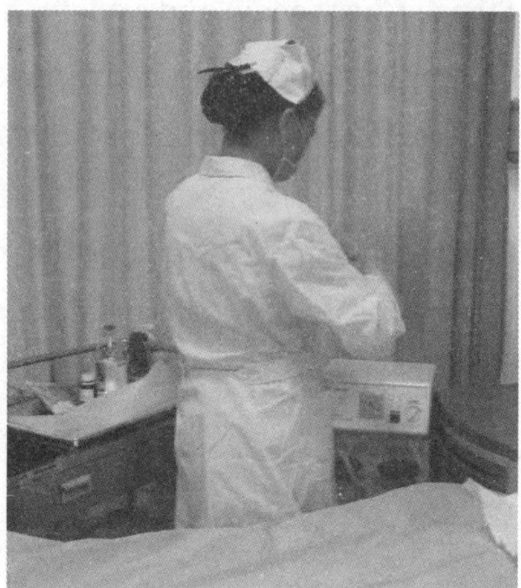
Connect Suction Tubing

Step 3: Suction.

- Suction small normal saline solution from basin.
- Insert catheter into mouth along gum line to pharynx. Replace oxygen mask.
- Rinse catheter with water in cup or basin until connecting tubing is cleared of secretions. Turn off suction. Wash face if secretions are present on the patient's skin.
- When suctioning is completed, roll catheter around fingers of dominant hand. Pull glove

off inside out so that catheter remains coiled in glove. Pull off other glove over first glove in the same way to seal in contaminants. Discard in contaminated waste receptacle. Turn off suction device.

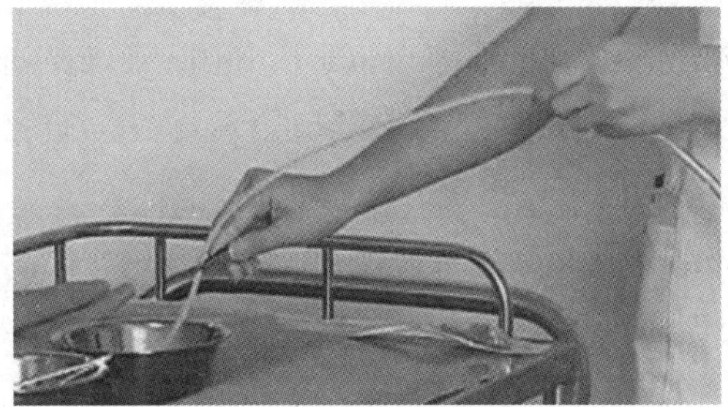

Suctioning

Step 4: Wind up.

- Remove towel, place in appropriate receptacle, and reposition the patient.
- Remove and discard face shield, and wash hands.
- Place unopened suction kit on suction machine or at head of bed according to institution preference.
- Compare the patient's respiratory assessments before and after suction.
- Ask the patient if breathing is easier and if congestion is decreased.
- Observe airway secretions.

Words and Phrases

suctioning	吸痰术	nasotracheal	鼻气管的
cannula	套管	orotracheal	口腔气管的
ventilation	通气	vomitus	呕吐物
perfusion	灌注	hypercapnia	血碳酸过多症
haemoglobin	血红蛋白	lethargy	嗜睡
molecule	分子	dysrhythmias	心律失常
oxyhaemoglobin	氧合血红蛋白	pallor	苍白
carbon dioxide	二氧化碳	cyanosis	发绀
nares	鼻孔	dyspnea	呼吸困难
elastic	有弹性的		

Learning Activities

Part I Choose the best answer for each question.

1. A patient is admitted to the emergency room in severe emotional distress. The patient's respirations are 42 times/min, and the blood gases reveal a pH of 7.5 and a $PaCO_2$ of 34. Initially the nurse should _______

A. instruct the client to breathe into a paper bag.

B. start an IV of D5W.

C. administer O_2 .

D. have the patient place his head between his knees.

2. The physician orders an arterial blood gas (ABG) for a patient receiving oxygen at 6 L/min. What information concerning the patient is most important for the nurse to document on the lab slip that accompanies the blood sample? _______

A. The patient's position in bed and the respiratory rate.

B. The site used to obtain the blood specimen.

C. The use of supplemental oxygen.

D. The patient's diagnosis and blood type.

3. The nurse is caring for a patient after a bronchoscopy. Which of the following would be most concerned by the nurse? _______

A. Depressed gag reflex.

B. Sputum streaked with blood.

C. Tachypnea.

D. Complaints of a sore throat.

4. The nurse has just returned to the desk and has four phone messages to return. Which of the following messages should the nurse return first? _______

A. A man with swelling of his left wrist following a fall from a ladder two hours ago.

B. A woman who had a cholecystectomy one week ago and now complains of redness and tenderness at the incision site.

C. A mother of a child reports that her son's lips are swollen following a fire ant bite.

D. A man with COPD reports he is coughing up large amounts of green-tinged sputum and has a temperature of 101.2 °F (38.4 °C).

5. The nurse is caring for a patient with pneumonia. Which of the following nursing observations would indicate a therapeutic response to the treatment? _______

A. Oral temperature of 101 °F (38.3 °C), increased chest pain with nonproductive cough.

B. Cough, productive of thick green sputum, client reports feeling tired.

C. Respirations at 20 times/min with no complaints of dyspnea, moderate amount of thin white sputum.

D. White cell count of 10,000 mm^3, urine output at 40 cc per hour, decreasing amount of sputum.

6. A 28-year-old woman at 39 weeks gestation in active labor screams, "I have to push, I have to push." The nurse notes that the patient is 8 cm dilated. The nurse should _______

A. instruct the patient to take a deep breath and bear down.

B. apply gentle but firm fundal pressure to the patient's abdomen.

C. coach the patient in relaxation techniques.

D. tell the patient to pant with pursed lips.

7. A patient has a Sengstaken-Blakemore tube in place. The nurse enters the room and finds the woman in respiratory distress. It is most important for the nurse to _______

A. notify the physician immediately to remove the tube.

B. elevate the head of the bed and administer oxygen.

C. cut the balloon ports and remove the tube.

D. call a code and begin rescue breathing.

8. Two days after admission, a patient's sputum culture is reported as positive for tuberculosis. While awaiting orders from the physician, the nurse should _______

A. initiate measures to transfer the client to a tuberculosis unit.

B. institute measures to initiate airborne precautions.

C. arrange for all of the patient's personal effects to be decontaminated.

D. notify the patirnt's family that they have been exposed to a contagious disease.

Part II Case study.

Case Scenario

A 75-year-old female patient, is admitted as pneumonia. When the patient comes to the hospital, her respiratory is 43 times/min, and lung auscultation has phlegmy sound. She is unable to cough up, and is oral bleeding. Apply oxygen and suction according to doctor's order.

Task: As her primary nurse, what should you do for this patient?

（郭玲玲　葛　炜）

Scenario Six

Gynecology and Pediatrics Nursing

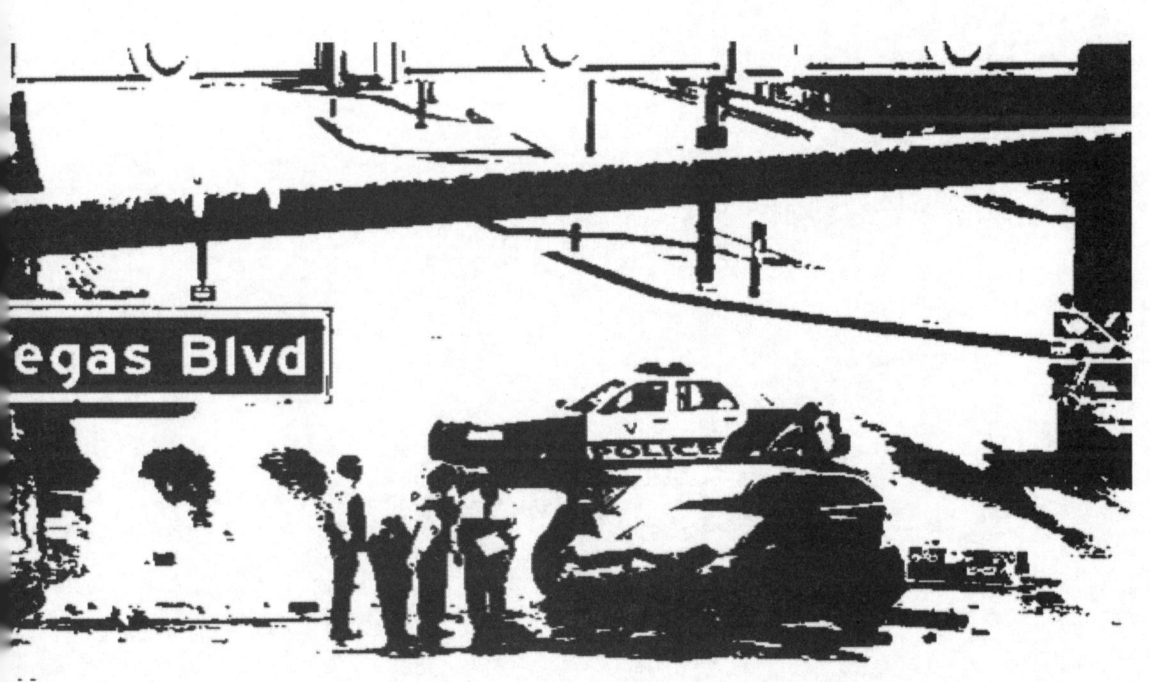

TASK
10 Maternal Abdominal Examination

Learning Outcomes

This task will provide students with opportunities to:

- Understand the purpose and importance of maternal abdominal examination.
- Master maternal abdominal examination.
- Communicate with pregnant women or others, write maternal healthcare card, and carry on the guidance and health education of pregnant women.

Scenario

Catherine is 32-year-old, 24 weeks of pregnancy. Her husband Bob accompanied with her to the hospital for prenatal examination. Also they brought their daughter Lucy for a growth assessment. Unfortunately, they were all involved in the car accident.

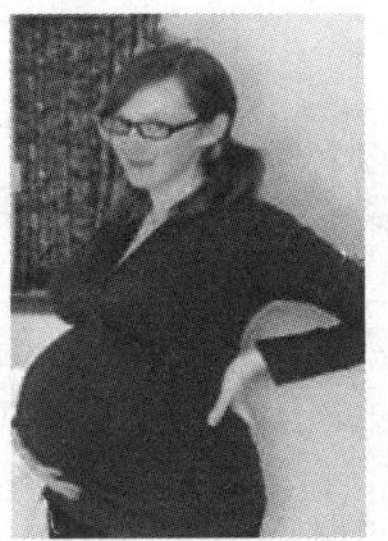

10-1 Maternal Abdominal Examination PPT

Background

Pregnant women should establish the perinatal health care card in 12 weeks of gestation, and do the first examination (body weight, blood pressure, blood routine, urine routine, and general physical examination). A series of prenatal examination begins in 20 weeks of pregnancy. During pregnancy 20 to 36 weeks, inspection needs to be done once every 4 weeks. From 36 weeks of gestation, inspection is conducted once every 1 week, i.e. 20, 24, 28, 32, 36, 37, 38, 39, 40 week each check 1 time, a total of 9 times. All high-risk pregnancy, should be appropriate to increase the inspection frequency. Maternal abdominal examination is an important part of the prenatal examination. It can help us to understand the development situation of the fetus, fetal lie, fetal position, and fetal heart sound. And it is useful for guidance and health education of pregnant women during pregnancy.

Category of Fetal Lie

1. Longitudinal lie: The ordinate axis between fetus and pregnant woman is parallel. This is the typical case for about 99.75% of pregnant women.

2. Transverse lie: The ordinate axis of fetal body is perpendicular to that of its mother, only 0.25% of pregnancy belongs to transverse lie.

3. Oblique lie: This case is normally temporary, and it would mostly develop into a longitudinal lie later, or in a rare case, it turns into a transverse lie.

Fetal Position

Fetal position is the position of the fetus in the uterus. Normal fetal position is the LOA and ROA.

10-2 Maternal Abdominal Examination 讲解视频

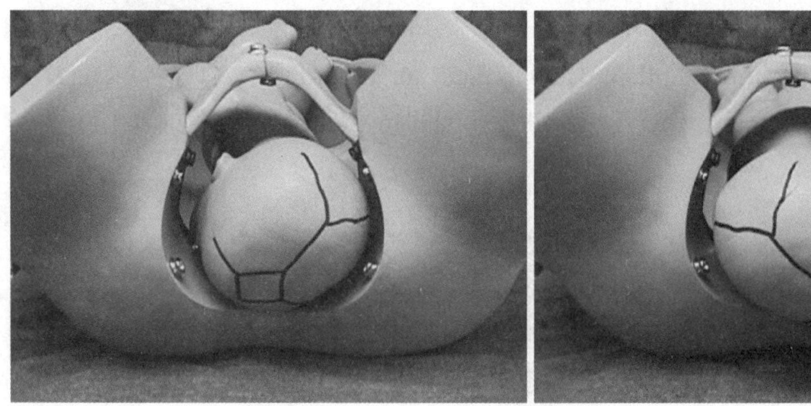

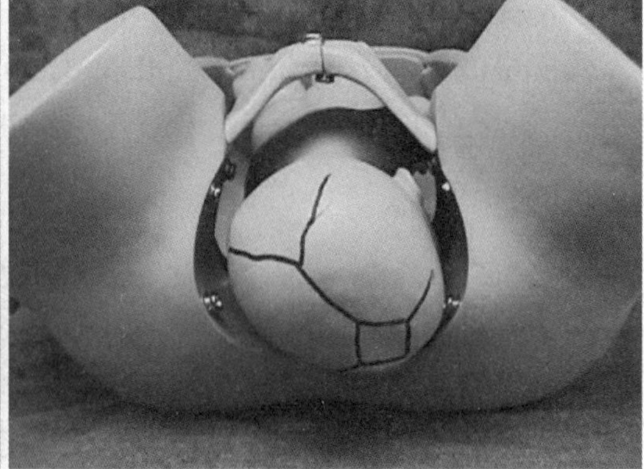

10-3 Maternal Abdominal Examination 操作视频

Procedure

Step1: Preparation before operation.

□ Pay attention to the protection of privacy and the environmental temperature.

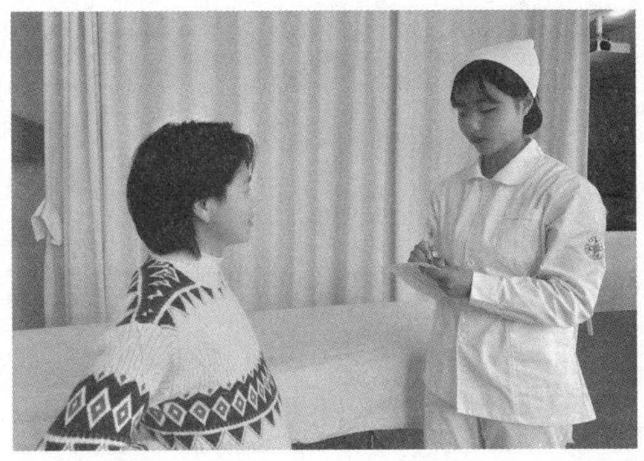

"Catherine, would you please put your maternal health care card to me? Before the examination, you'll have to go to urinate."

Step 2: Inspection.

□ Observe the abdominal shape, size, stretch marks, scars, venous engorgement, edema.

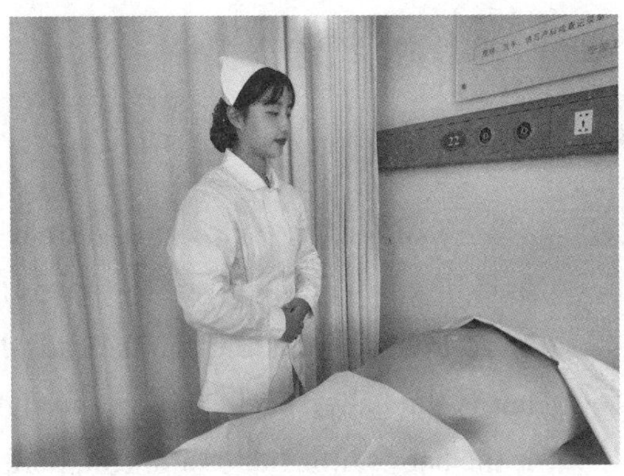

"Catherine, your abdomen size is pregnant in six months, oval, no striae gravidarum, no edema, no operation scar, no varices."

Step 3: Measuring uterine fundal height.

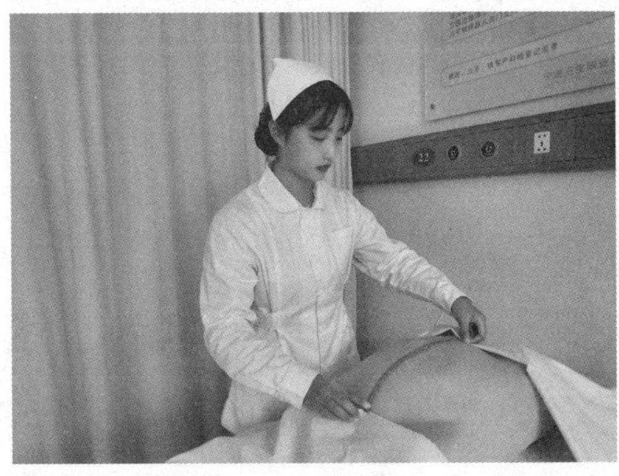

"Your uterine fundal height is 24 cm."

Step 4: Measuring abdominal circumference.

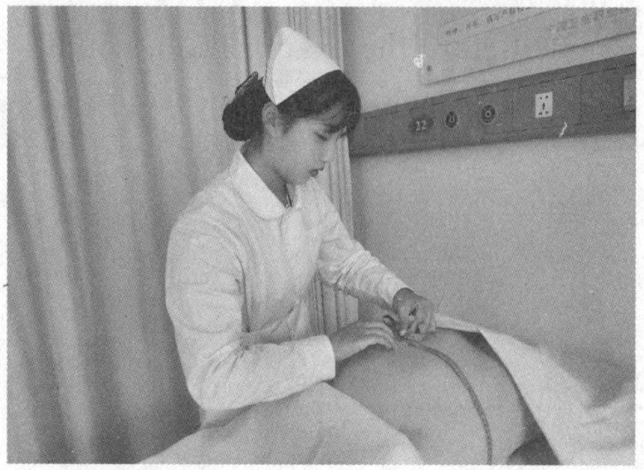

"Your abdominal circumference is 78 cm. "

Step5: Four maneuvers of Leopold.

□ Check the uterine size, fetal lie, fetal presentation, and fetal position.

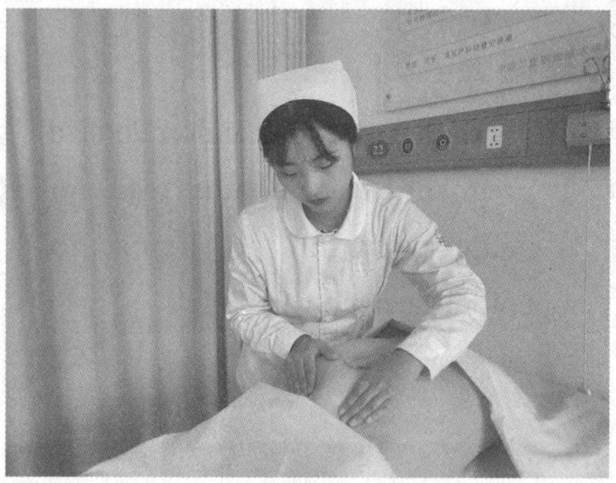

"Catherine, please put your legs buckling up. I'll help you to touch the baby. Look, here is the baby's head, the left is the baby's back, and on the right is the baby's little hands and feet, here is the baby's little ass."

Step 6: Auscultation.

□ Put the stethoscope on the fetal dorsal.

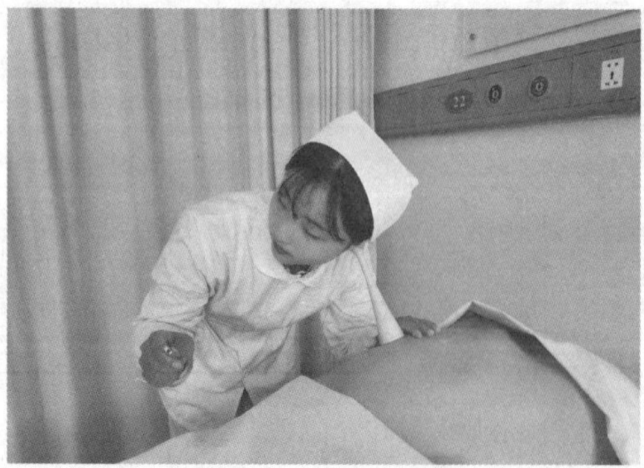

"The baby's heart rate is 140 bpm."

Step 7: Recording the checking results.

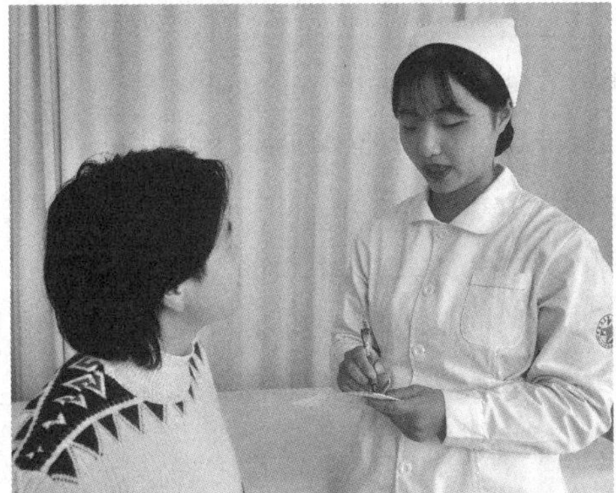

"Catherine, your examination results are normal. You should pay attention to a balanced diet. If you have any abnormal symptoms, come to the hospital in time. Don't forget to check next month."

Words and Phrases

urinate	排尿	fetal presentation	胎先露
symptom	症状	fetal position	胎方位
spmptomatic	症状的	four maneuvers of leopold	四步触诊法
fetal lie	胎产式		

Learning Activities

Part I Choose the best answer for each question.

1. A 28-year-old client delivered a full-term male neonate one hour ago. Which finding should the nurse expect when palpating the client's fundus? ________

A. Soft, at the level of the umbilicus.

B. Firm, 2 cm below the umbilicus.

C. Firm, at the level of the umbilicus.

D. Boggy, midway between the umbilicus and symphysis pubis.

2. A 34-year-old client is 34 weeks pregnant and is experiencing bleeding caused by placenta previa. The fetal heart sounds are normal and the client isn't in labor. Which of the following nursing interventions should be of priority? ________

A. Monitor the amount of vaginal blood loss.

B. Allow the client to ambulate with assistance.

C. Perform a vaginal examination to check for cervical dilation.

D. Notify the physician for a fetal heart rate of 130 beats/minute.

3. A 24-year-old primipara decides to breast-feed her baby but says, "I am worried

that I won't be able to breast-feed my baby because my breasts are so small." Which of the following is appropriate response by the nurse? ________

A. Because her breasts are small, she will have to feed the baby more often.

B. Breast size poses no influence on a woman's ability to breast-feed a baby.

C. Breast milk can be enhanced by occasional formula feeding.

D. The woman's motivation to breast-feed is less important than breast size.

4. A 30-year-old client with 7 months pregnancy reports severe leg cramps at night. Which nursing action would be most effective in helping her cope with these cramps? ____

A. Suggesting that she walk for l hour twice per day.

B. Advismg her to take over-the-counter calcium supplements twice per day.

C. Teaching her to dorsiflex her foot during the cramp.

D. Instructing her to increase milk and cheese intake to 8 to 10 servings per day.

5. A multigravid client in active labor is about to deliver. The nurse has no help immediately available. What should the nurse do first? ________

A. Prepare a clean area on which to deliver the neonate.

B. Lower the head of the bed to a flat position.

C. Have the client push with a contraction.

D. Ask the client to take a deep breath and hold it.

6. The client delivers a viable male neonate who is given a score of 9 at the fifth minute after born on the Apgar rating system. The client asks the nurse what it means. The nurse interprets this finding as indicating that the neonate's physical condition is ________.

A. good　　B. fair

C. poor　　D. critical

7. Mrs. Wilson, a primigravida, was admitted to the hospital at 12 weeks' gestation. She is complaining of abdominal cramping and exhibiting bright red spotting in vagina without cervical dilation. Which of the following types of abortion does the nurse determine that the client is most likely experiencing? ________.

A. Complete　　B. Threatened

C. Inevitable　　D. Missed

8. A multigravida at 37 week's gestation tells the nurse that she has frequent heartburn. The nurse teaches the client with suggestions for obtaining relief from the heartburn. Which of the following statements made by the patient indicates that she has understood the nurse's instructions? ________

A."I can take a teaspoon of baking soda in water occasionally."

B."I should eat only three large meals and drink plenty of fluids."

C."It's all right for me to have a fried hamburger and fries."

D."I should eat smaller, more frequent meals with fluids."

9. A 34-year-old client is 34 weeks pregnant and is experiencing bleeding caused by placenta previa. The fetal heart sounds are normal and the client isn't in labor. Which of the following nursing interventions should be of priority? ________

A. Monitor the amount of vaginal blood loss.

B. Allow the client to ambulate with assistance.

C. Perform a vaginal examination to check for cervical dilation.

D. Notify the physician for a fetal heart rate of 130 beats/min.

10. The nurse is teaching a client who is 28 weeks pregnant and has gestational diabetes how to control her blood glucose level. Diet therapy alone has been unsuccessful in controlling this client's blood glucose level, so she has started insulin therapy. Which of the following statements indicates the client has adequate knowledge? ________

A. "I won't use insulin if I'm sick."

B. "I need to use insulin each day."

C. "If I give myself an insulin injection, I don't need to watch what I eat."

D. "I'll monitor my blood glucose level twice a week."

11. A nurse in a prenatal clinic is assessing a 28-year-old woman who is 24 weeks pregnant. Which of the following findings would lead this nurse to suspect that the client has mild preeclampsia? ________

A. Hypertension, edema, proteinuria.

B. Glycosuria, hypertension, seizures.

C. Hematuria, blurry vision, reduced urine output.

D. Burning on urination, hypotension, abdominal pain.

Part II Case study.

Case Scenario

Sarah is a 28-year-old multigravida. She has a 5-year-old girl and a 2-year-old boy. This is her third pregnancy. Now she is 37 weeks pregnant. She complains about the hemorrhoidal pain and the blood pressure is 160/110 mmHg.

Task: Carry on the guidance and health education.

（梅一宁　吴珊珊）

TASK 11 Growth and Development

Learning Outcomes

This task will provide students with opportunities to:

- Understand relative implication of physical indicators in growth and development.
- Measure and record important physical indicators for children precisely.
- Assess the growth of the child and provide appropriate guidance for parents.

Scenario

Lucy is a 3-month-old baby who was unfortunately involved in the car accident with her mother. She was immediately delivered to the pediatric department for body check-up. Fortunately, Lucy was put in the safety seat and didn't get hurt.

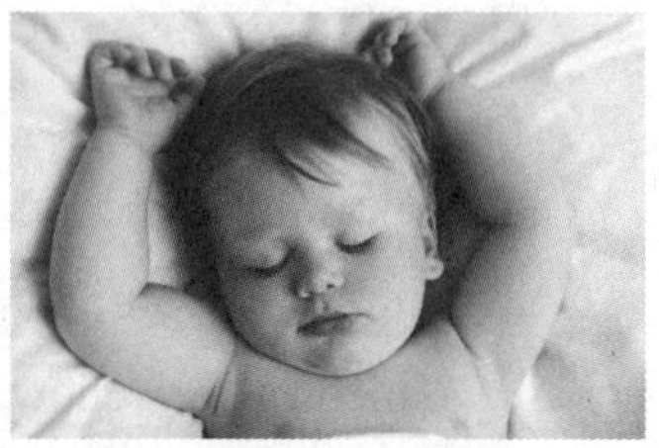

11-1 Growth and Development PPT

Background

From the moment parents greet their newborn, they watch the baby's progress eagerly, anticipating every inch of growth and each new developmental milestone along the way. To make sure their babies grow properly, some physical indicators are used to indicate and assess the pace of the growth.

Physical growth refers to the increases in height and weight and other body changes that occur as a child matures. Hair grows; teeth come in, come out, and come in again; and eventually puberty hits. It's all part of the growth process.

The first year of life is a time of astonishing change during which babies, on average, grow 10 inches (25 cm) in length and triple their birth weights.

After birth, the height of baby grows slowly from the first year to the second year. After 2 years old, the growth in height usually continues at a fairly steady rate of approximately 2.5

inches (6 cm) per year until adolescence.

To help parents recognize the normal growth range, BMI and growth chart are developed by pediatricians.

BMI (Body Mass Index)

BMI is a formula that doctors use to estimate how much body fat a person has based on his or her weight and height. The BMI formula uses height and weight measurements to calculate a BMI number. Though the formula is the same for adults and children, figuring out what the BMI number means is a little more complicated for kids.

For kids, BMI is plotted on a growth chart that uses percentile lines to tell whether a child is underweight, healthy weight, overweight, or obese. Different BMI charts are used for boys and girls under the age of 20 because the amount of body fat differs between boys and girls and body fat changes as kids grow.

Each BMI chart is divided into percentiles. A child whose BMI is equal to or greater than the 5th percentile and less than the 85th percentile is considered a healthy weight for his or her age. If the BMI is at or above the 85th percentile but less than the 95th percentile, it is considered as overweight. The BMI at or above the 95th percentile is considered as obese. The BMI below the 5th percentile is considered as underweight.

Before you calculate your child's BMI, you'll need an accurate height and weight measurement. Bathroom scales and tape measures aren't always precise. So the best way to get accurate measurements is by having kids weighed and measured at a doctor's office or at school.

You can calculate BMI on your own, but consider asking your doctor to help you figure out what it means. Doctors do more than just use BMI to assess a child's current weight. They also take into account where a child is during puberty and use BMI results from past years to track whether that child may be at risk for becoming overweight. Spotting this risk early on can be helpful because changes can be made before developing a weight problem.

Kids are developing weight-related health problems previously seen only in adults. Type 2 diabetes, high cholesterol, and high blood pressure are now commonly seen in overweight and obese kids and teens. They're also more likely to be overweight as adults. And adults who are overweight may develop other serious health conditions, such as heart disease.

Although BMI can be a good indicator of body fat, it doesn't always tell the full story. Someone with a large frame or a lot of muscle instead of excess fat (like a bodybuilder or athlete) can have a high BMI. Likewise, a small person with a small frame may have a normal BMI but could still have too much body fat. These are other good reasons to talk about your BMI with your doctor.

Growth Chart

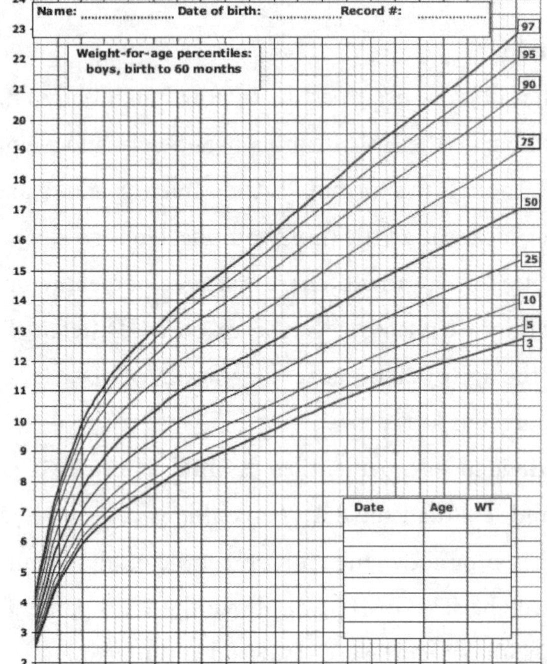

Boys' Weight-for-age Growth Chart

Growth charts are a standard part of any checkup, and they show health care providers how kids are growing compared with other kids of the same age and gender. They also allow doctors and nurses to see the pattern of kids' height and weight gain over time, and whether they're developing proportionately.

A child was growing along the same pattern until he was 2 years old, then suddenly started growing at a much slower rate than other kids. That might indicate a health problem. Doctors could see that by looking at a growth chart.

Not everyone grows and develops on the same schedule. During puberty, the body begins making hormones that spark physical changes like breast development in girls and testicular enlargement in boys and spurts in height and weight gain in both boys and girls. Once these changes start, they continue for several years. The average person can expect to grow as much as 10 inches (25 cm) during puberty before reaching full adult height.

Most kids gain weight more rapidly during this time as the amounts of muscle, fat, and bone in their bodies change. All that new weight gain can be perfectly fine—as long as body fat, muscle, and bone are in the right proportion.

Because some kids start developing as early as age 8 and some not until age 14, it can be normal for two kids who are the same gender, height, and age to have very different weights.

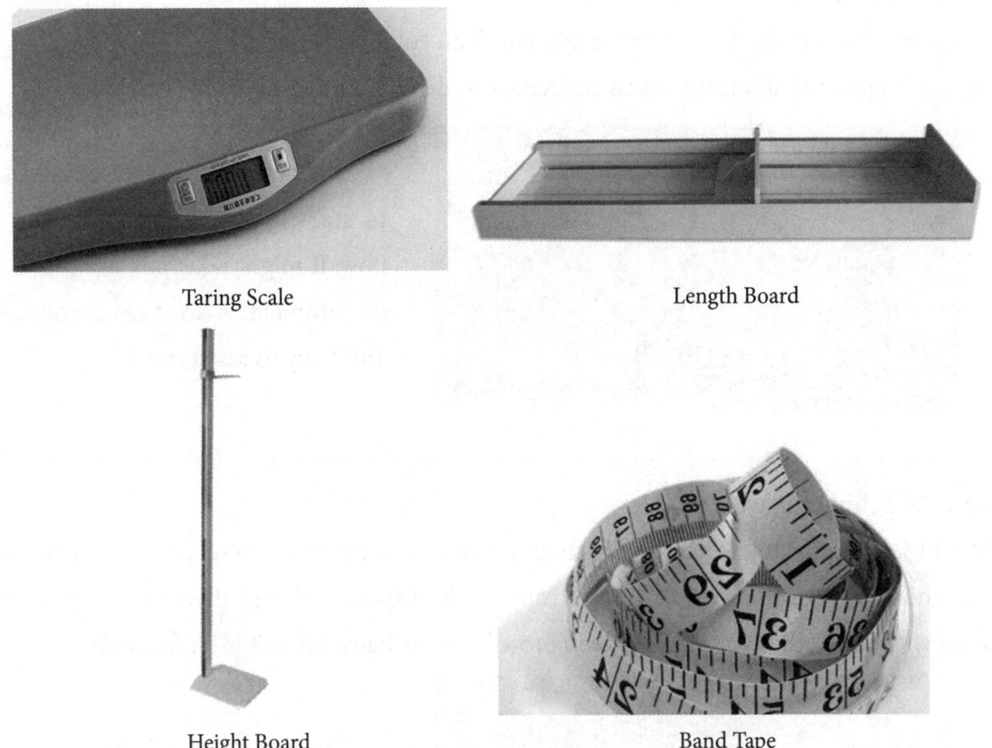

Taring Scale

Length Board

Height Board

Band Tape

You may need these equipment in the assessment:

- A taring scale.
- A length board or a height board.
- A band tape.
- Paper towels or soft clothes to cover the length/height board.
- Small toys or fruit to entertain the children and offer to take home.
- Several cups and bowls to show quantities of food servings for children.
- Small toys to entertain the children and offer as presents to take home.
- If possible, thank for the parents, such as a gift certificate for groceries.

11-2 Growth and Development 讲解视频

Procedure

Step 1: Preparation before assessment.

▫ Warm the room to 26 ℃ in advance and check all equipment.

▫ Explain to parents about the assess procedure and get their assistance.

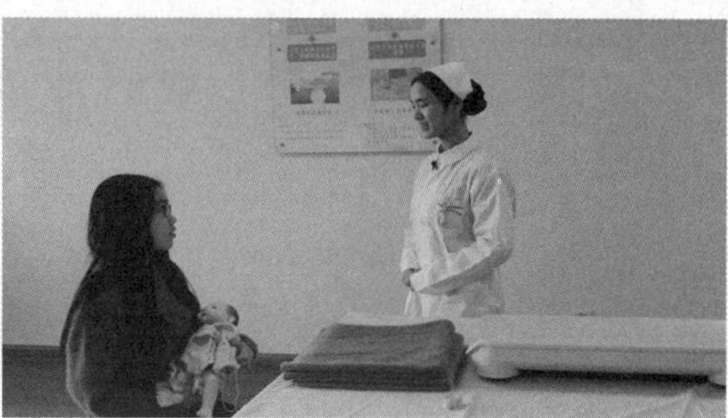

"Catherine, we are going to start the assess procedure now. It might take half an hour to complete. Also, I need you and Lucy to assist me."

Step 2: Weighing the weight.

▫ Weight is an indicator which implies baby's nutrition level. Put a towel on the taring scale and then turn on the scale. The electronic scale displays "0" and then put Lucy on the scale without clothes and diaper. Keep protecting the baby when it is on the scale.

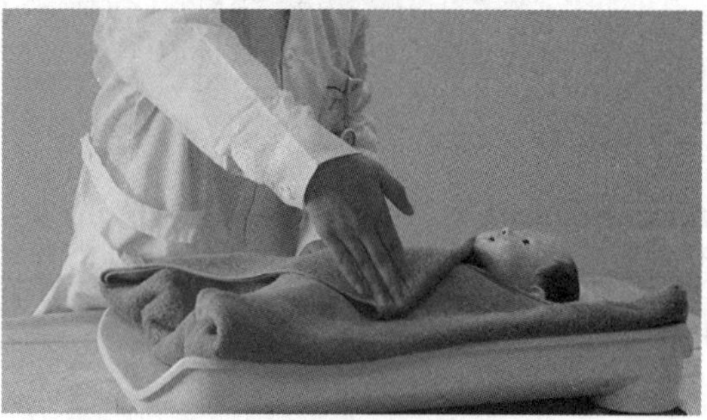

"Lucy's weight is 5.5 kilograms now. It is quiet appropriate for her age. Catherine, you really feed her well."

Step 3: Measuring the baby's length/height.

▫ Length/Height describes the growth of bones. Measure the baby in a supine position on the length board until 3 years old. Make sure the baby's legs straight during the procedure.

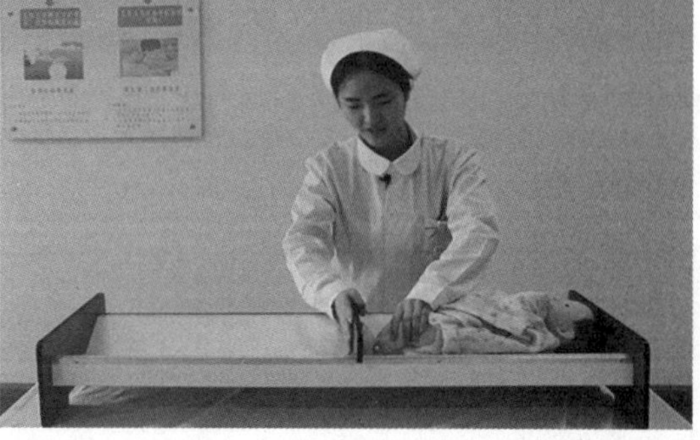

"She is 60 centimeters long. Her bones grow rapidly in this period. Add Vitamin D and take her to join in activities outside."

Step 4: Measuring sitting length/height.

▫ Sitting height implies part of the bone growth. It is from the roof of head to the bottom.

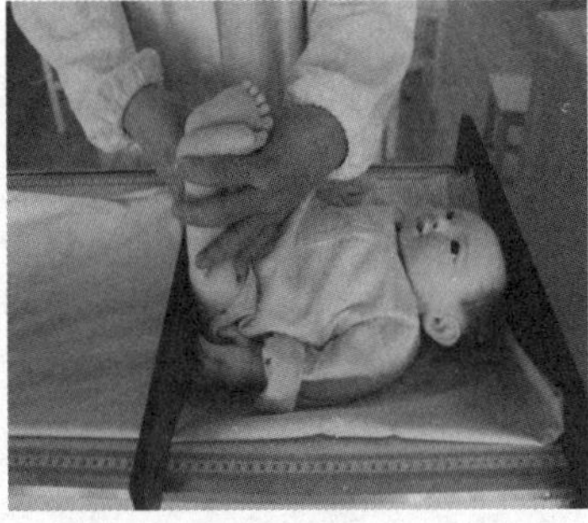

"Her sitting length is 42 cm. It is average."

Step 5: Measuring head circumference.

▫ This circumference indicates the growth of skull and brain. The average head circumference is about 34 cm at birth.

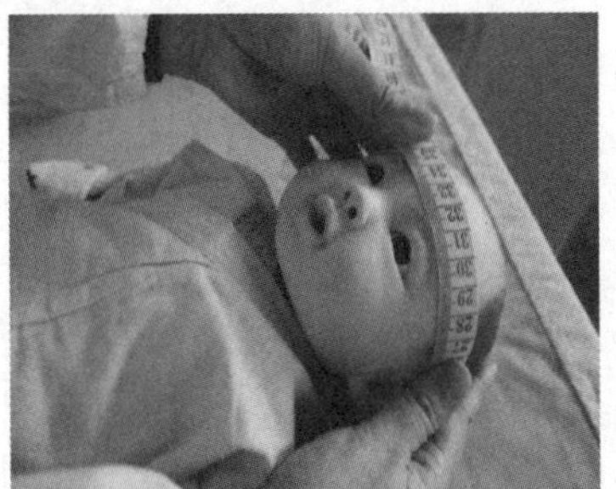

"Head circumference is 34 cm now. Lucy is smart."

Step 6: Measuring chest circumference.

▫ Chest circumference describes the growth of lung, chest fat, and also the pattern of the chest. It is about 32 cm at birth. It remains smaller than head circumference until 1 year old.

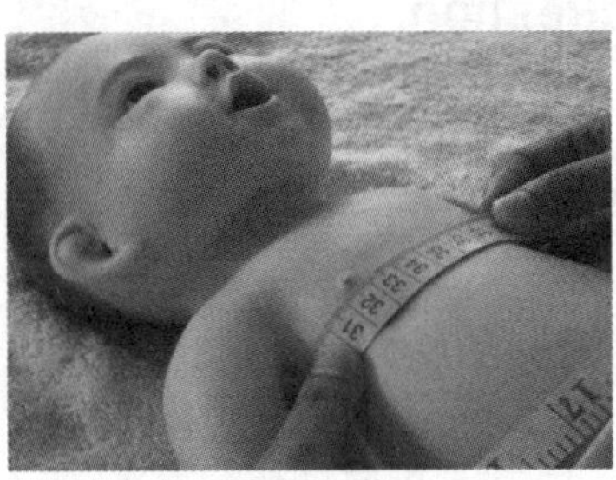

"We have to measure it twice respectively in the beginning and ending of the breath. And we record the average number as a final chest circumference. Lucy's chest circumference is 32 cm. It's pretty good."

Step 7: Recording all results and draw a conclusion.

▫ After measuring all indicators, nurses should draw a conclusion about the physical growth as a whole. Explain to parents about all results and provide relative guidance to promote the growth.

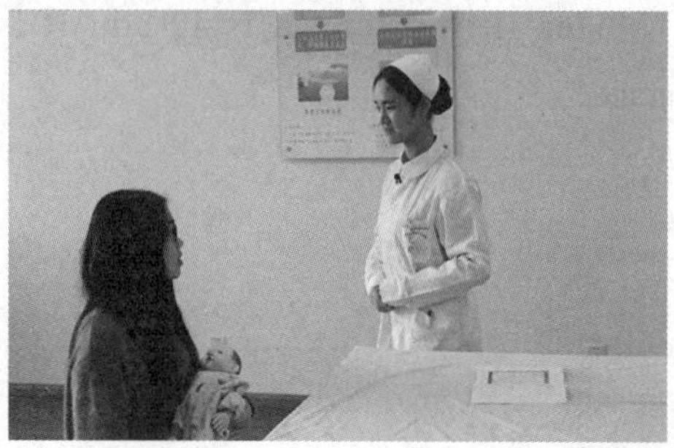

"Catherine, all indicators showed Lucy is under a good physical growth. Thank you for your cooperation. "

11-3 Growth and Development 操作视频

Words

circumference	周长	diaper	尿布
indicator	指标	imply	说明；表明
taring	去皮的		

Learning Activities

Part I Choose the best answer for each question.

1. A nurse is teaching the parents of a 6-month-old infant about usual growth and development. Which statement about infant development is true? ________

A. A 6-month-old infant has difficulty holding objects.

B. A 6-month-old infant can usually roll from prone to supine and supine to prone position.

C. Stranger anxiety usually peaks at age 12 to 18 months.

D. The infant's head circumference is smaller than chest circumference.

2. Before a well checkup in the pediatrician's office, an 8-month-old infant is sitting contentedly on the mother's lap, chewing a toy. When preparing to examine this infant,

which step should the nurse do first? ________

A. Obtain body weight.

B. Auscultate heart and breath sounds.

C. Check papillary response.

D. Measure the head circumference.

3. A mother brings her infant to the pediatrician's office for his 2-week-old check-up. The nurse is evaluating whether the mother has understood teaching points discussed during a previous visit. Which statement indicates that further teaching is needed? ________

A. "I don't understand why my baby doesn't look at me."

B. "I know I should keep my baby's nasal passages clear."

C. "I should limit my baby's exposure during bath time."

D. "I should cover my baby's head when he's wet or cold."

4. A nurse is teaching the parents of a school-age child. Which teaching topic should take priority? ________

A. Accident prevention.

B. Keeping a night light on to allay fears.

C. Normalcy of fears about body integrity.

D. Encouraging the child to dress without help.

5. A nurse is evaluating the developmental level of a 2-year-old child. Which of the following does the nurse expect to observe in this child? ________

A. Uses a fork to eat.

B. Uses a cup to drink.

C. Pours own milk into a cup.

D. Uses a knife for cutting food.

6. A 2-year-old child is treated in the emergency room for a burn to the chest and abdomen. The child sustained the burn by grabbing a cup of hot coffee that was left on the kitchen counter. The nurse reviews safety principles with the parents before discharge. Which statement made by the parents indicates an understanding of measures to provide safety in the home? ________

A. "We will be sure not to leave hot liquids unattended."

B. "I guess my children need to understand what the word hot means."

C. "We will be sure that the children stay in their rooms when we work in the kitchen."

D. "We will install a safety gate as soon as we get home so the children cannot get into the kitchen."

7. A mother arrives at a clinic with her toddler and tells a nurse that she has a difficult time getting the child to go to bed at night. Which of the following is appropriate for the

nurse to suggest to the mother? ________

A. Avoid a nap during the day.

B. Allow the child to set bedtime limits.

C. Allow the child to have temper tantrums.

D. Inform the child of bedtime a few minutes before it is time for bed.

8. A mother of a 3-year-old child asks a clinic nurse about appropriate and safe toys for the child. The nurse tells the mother that the most appropriate toy for a 3-year-old child is ________.

A. a wagon

B. a golf set

C. a farm set

D. a jack set with marbles

9. A nurse is preparing to care for a 5-year-old child who has been placed in traction following a fracture of the femur. The nurse plans care, knowing that ________ is most appropriate for this child.

A. a radio

B. a sports video

C. large picture books

D. crayons and a coloring book

Part II Case study.

Case Scenario

Mike is a 10-month-old infant. He was delivered at only 28 gestational weeks. Now he is 6 kg heavy and 65 centimeters long.

Task: Please evaluate Mike's physical growth and provide appropriate guidance for his parents in feeding.

（吴珊珊　梅一宁）

Appendix

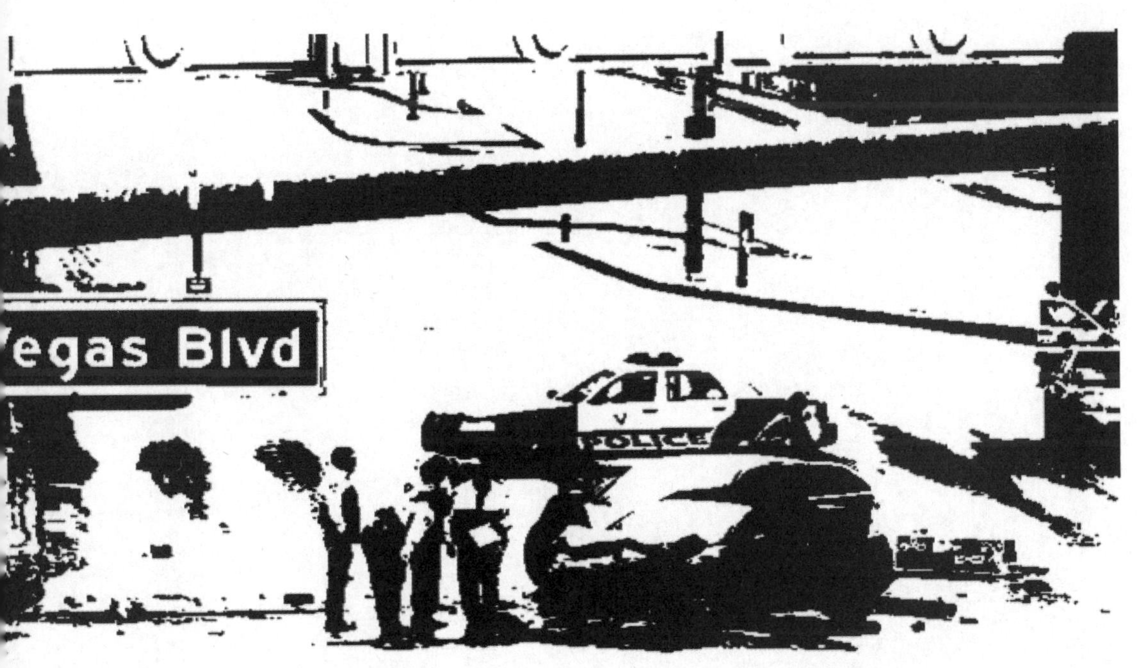

Appendix 1 Hospital Admission Form

Patient Admission Form

IMPORTANT: Please send this completed form to the Hospital where you will have your procedure/surgery.

PERSONAL AND ADMINISTRATION DETAILS

Surname (family name): ________________ Mr☐ Mrs☐ Ms☐ Miss☐ Mstr☐ Dr☐

First name(s): ________________ **Preferred name:** ________________

Date of birth: ____/____/____ (d m y) **Gender:** Male☐ Female☐ **NHI:** ________________

Residential address: ________________

Postal address: ________________

Email address: ________________

Telephone: (Home) ________ (Business) ________ (Mobile) ________

New Zealand resident: Yes☐ No☐

Ethnicity: European / Maori / Pacific Island / Asian / Middle Eastern / Latin American / African / Other ________
Please circle one or more

General Practitioner: ________________ **Telephone:** ________________

NEXT OF KIN/CONTACT PERSON

Name: ________________ **Relationship to patient:** ________________

Address: ________________

Telephone: (Home) ________ (Business) ________ (Mobile) ________

PAYMENT DETAILS

How will your procedure be paid for? Tick and complete as many as applies:

☐ **Health insurance** (personal expenses such as telephone calls may be excluded)

Insurance details: ________________ Membership No: ________________

Have you obtained "prior approval" for payment? Yes☐ No☐ Approval No: ________________

☐ **ACC** (personal expenses such as telephone calls are excluded)

☐ **Paid personally** If you are paying for the procedure yourself, please note that some procedures may require a deposit before admission. Your Shurgeon's rooms or hospital may inform you if a deppsit applies.

ACCOUNT SETTLEMENT AND CREDIT CARD AUTHORISATION

I will pay my account by: Cheque☐ Cash☐ Credit card☐ Eftpos☐

If you select credit card as your payment option, please complete and sign:

Card type: MasterCard☐ Visa☐ Diners☐ AMEX☐

Credit card number: ☐☐☐☐ ☐☐☐☐ ☐☐☐☐ ☐☐☐☐ Expiry date: ____/____ (m y)

Name on credit card: ________________ Signature: ________________

I understand that signing this Credit Card Authority authorises Southern Cross Hospital to debit my credit card with all amounts due and owing to Southern Cross Hospital in relation to my admission and treatment at Southern Cross Hospital on date: ____/____/____ (d m y)

AGREEMENT

I agree to settle my Hospital account in full at the time of my discharge when personally paying my account or where I do not have "prior approval" from my insurer. I understand I am responsible for any outstanding balance if my procedure is not fully covered by insurance, ACC or other contract. I give permission for Southern Cross to obtain any information relating to the approval/claim for this admission from the relevant funder/s, and I authorise that person or organisation to disclose such information to Southern Cross Hospital. I accept that, in the event my Hospital account is not met, Southern Cross reserves the right to add all costs of collection to this account. I give permission to Southern Cross Hospital or any health professional involved in my care for this admission to Hospital, to access health information about me that is relevant to my current treatment, which may be held by Southern Cross, other health professionals or other health organisations. I understand the admitting Surgeon, Anaesthetist and other Doctors or health professionals using Southern Cross facilities are independent and not employees of Southern Cross, with respect to both my treatment, care and account payment. I accept that this agreement is covered by New Zealand law.

The details above have been completed by:

Name: ________________ Date: ____/____/____ (d m y)

Signature: ________________

If not the patient, state relationship to patient: ________________

Appendix 2 Surgical Consent Form

PATIENT CONSENT TO PROCEDURE PATIENT: UNIT NO: PROCEDURE: ☒Right ☒Left ☒Both Sides ☒Not applicable	

I understand my illness/medical condition and the procedure/surgery I will be having. I understand the risks and benefits i can reasonably expect from this procedure/surgery, compared to those i could expect from other approaches

I understand the risks and the possibility of major complications of this procedure/surgery. I understand that among the risks of this procedure are drug reactions, bleeding, infection, and complications from receiving blood or blood components. I also understand that, as with every procedure/surgery, there is the possibility of unexpected complicat ions

The following additional specific risks or issues were discussed with me: **[Physician/Licensed Practitioner, please list]**

☒I received teaching materials to help me understand the information explained to me.

☒Procedural sedation will be used during this procedure/surgery to control my pain. I understand that this method of pain control has risks, including the possibility of suppressed breathing, low blood pressure and, sometimes, incomplete pain relief.

Doctor________________________________will perform my procedure/surgery.

I understand that Massachusetts General Hospital (MGH) is a teaching hospital. This means that resident doctors, doctors in medical fellowships (fellows) and students in medical, nursing, and related health care professions receive training here. These doctors and students may take part in my procedure/surgery. My doctor will determine when it is necessary or appropriate for others to participate in my procedure/surgery and care.

I understand that th is procedure/surgery may have significant educational or scientific value. The hospital may photograph, videotape, or record my procedure/surgery for teaching purposes. Any information used for these purposes will not identify me I understand that blood or other samples removed to treat or diagnose my condition may later be thrown away by MGH. Those materials also may be used by MGH, by medical organizations connected to MGH, or by educational or business organizations approved by MGH, for research, education and other activities that support MGH's mission.

I have had an opportunity to ask about the risks and benefits of this procedure/surgery and of the alternatives. All my questions have been answered to my satisfaction, and I consent to this procedure/surgery:

Date______________Time______________AM/PM__________________

Signature (patient/health care agent/guardian/family member) (I f patient's consent cannot be obtained, indicate reason above.)

lattest that I discussed all relevant aspects of this procedure/surgery, including the indications, risks, and benefits, as compared with alternativo approaches, with the patient, and answered his/her questions.

Date______________Time______________AM/PM__________________

Signature (Physician/Licensed Practitioner) __________________

Appendix 3 Operating Criteria for Medical Care

<table>
<tr><th colspan="2">Project</th><th>Rules</th><th>Score</th></tr>
<tr><td rowspan="11">Practice
(40分)</td><td rowspan="2">Connect the monitor</td><td>Open the monitor</td><td>2</td></tr>
<tr><td>Connect the monitor to the client correctly</td><td>3</td></tr>
<tr><td rowspan="3">Oxygen</td><td>Select the right type of oxygen</td><td>2</td></tr>
<tr><td>Implement oxygen correctly</td><td>5</td></tr>
<tr><td>Adjust oxygen flow rate correctly</td><td>3</td></tr>
<tr><td rowspan="5">IV</td><td>Assess the illness, vein condition of client</td><td>2</td></tr>
<tr><td>Exhaust the air in the tube twice</td><td>4</td></tr>
<tr><td>Sterile the skin of puncture site correctly</td><td>6</td></tr>
<tr><td>Insert successfully</td><td>4</td></tr>
<tr><td>Fixed and adjust correctly</td><td>4</td></tr>
<tr><td>ECG</td><td>Observe ECG correctly</td><td>5</td></tr>
<tr><td colspan="2" rowspan="4">Communication (20分)</td><td>Word accurately</td><td>5</td></tr>
<tr><td>Language is fluent</td><td>5</td></tr>
<tr><td>Express clearly</td><td>5</td></tr>
<tr><td>Affinity</td><td>5</td></tr>
<tr><td colspan="2" rowspan="5">Recording (20分)</td><td>Connect the monitor (connect time and initial data)</td><td>4</td></tr>
<tr><td>Oxygen (time, flow rate and client's reaction)</td><td>4</td></tr>
<tr><td>IV (time, drop and client's reaction)</td><td>4</td></tr>
<tr><td>ECG</td><td>4</td></tr>
<tr><td>Others</td><td>4</td></tr>
<tr><td colspan="2" rowspan="3">Team work (20分)</td><td>The team leader command</td><td>6</td></tr>
<tr><td>Team members can follow leader's instructions</td><td>6</td></tr>
<tr><td>Solidarity and collaboration between all the team members</td><td>8</td></tr>
</table>

Evaluator: Time:

Appendix 4 Operating Criteria for Maternal Abdominal Examination

Project		Rules	Score
Practice (40分)	Preparation before operation	Prepare for material, placed reasonable	2
		Pay attention to the protection of privacy, pay attention to the environmental temperature	3
	Inspection	The narrative content integrity	5
	Measurement	Measuring uterine fundal height	5
		Measuring abdominal circumference	5
	Four maneuvers of Leopold	The first step	4
		The second step	4
		The third step	4
		The fourth step	4
	Auscultation	Accurate reading	4
Communication (20分)		Word accurately	5
		Language is fluent	5
		Express clearly	5
		affinity	5
Recording and health education (20分)		Fetal position	4
		Fetal presentation	4
		FHR(fetal heart rate)	4
		Fetal size	4
		Fetal lie	4
Team work (20分)		The team leader command	6
		Team members can follow leader's instructions	6
		Solidarity and collaboration between all the team members	8

Evaluator:　　　　Time:

Appendix 5 Operating Criteria for First Aid

Project		Rules	Score
Practice (40分)	Preparation before operation	Prepare for material	2
		Assess environment and determine consciousness	3
		Initiate EMSS	
	CPR	Do the CPR correctly	20
	Bleeding control	Choose the right site to stop bleeding. Mark it correctly.	4
	Dressing	Treat wounds correctly.	4
	Fixation	Methods of fixation is correct.	4
	Moving	Choose the suitable moving method	3
Communication (20分)		Word accurately	5
		Language is fluent	5
		Express clearly	5
		Emergency consciousness	5
Recording and health education (20分)		CPR (Record the emergency time, process, etc.)	10
		Trauma care (process)	10
Team work (20分)		The team leader command	6
		Team members can follow leader's instructions	6
		Solidarity and collaboration between all the team members	8

Evaluator: Time:

References

[1] 陈树宝 . 儿科学 [M]. 北京 : 北京科学出版社，2017.

[2] 崔红 . 医疗行业英语教程 [M]. 杭州 : 浙江大学出版社，2012.

[3] 费素定 . 基本救护技术 [M]. 杭州 : 浙江大学出版社，2020.

[4] 桂莉 .CGFNS 考试解析与实战模拟 [M]. 上海 : 上海科学技术出版社，2006.

[5] 姜丽萍 . 护理英语教程 [M]. 杭州 : 浙江大学出版社，2010.

[6] 姜学智 , 陈晓军 . 妇产科临床英语会话集 [M]. 北京 : 人民卫生出版社，2016.

[7] 李乐之 , 路潜 . 外科护理学 [M]. 北京 : 人民卫生出版社，2017.

[8] 李小寒 , 尚少梅 . 护理学基础 [M]. 北京 : 人民卫生出版社，2017.

[9] 美国护校毕业生国际委员会 . 国际护士执业水平考试（ISPN）官方指南 [M]. 中康（北京）人力资源管理中心 , 译 . 北京 : 高等教育出版社，2016.

[10] 王莘 . 医护英语水平考试（METS）指导与实训（第一级）[M]. 北京 : 人民卫生出版社，2013.

[11] 王莘 . 医护英语水平考试（METS）指导与实训（第二级）[M]. 北京 : 人民卫生出版社，2013.

[12] 王莘 . 医护英语水平考试（METS）指导与实训（第三级）[M]. 北京 : 人民卫生出版社，2013.

[13] 王文秀，王颖 . 英汉对照医务英语会话 [M]. 北京 : 人民卫生出版社，2016.

[14] 王文秀 , 王颖 . 护理英语会话 [M]. 北京 : 人民卫生出版社，2017.

[15] 徐小萍 , 刘佳 , 杨阳 . 妇产科护理实训指导 [M]. 北京 : 中国协和医科大学出版社，2019.

[16] 尤黎明 , 吴瑛 . 内科护理学 [M]. 北京 : 人民卫生出版社，2017.

[17] 朱琦 . 医学英语 [M]. 上海 : 上海交通大学出版社，2012.

[18] Amy M. Karach. Nursing Drug Guide[M]. Philadelphia: Lippincott Williams & Wilkins, 2001.

[19] Dav-Ellen Chabner. Medical Terminology—A Short Course [M]. 8th ed. Amsterdam: Elsevier-Health Sc，2020.

[20] Jennifer Fraser,Donna Waters, Elizabeth Forster, et al. Pediatric Nursing in Australia: Principles for practice[M]. London: Cambridge University Press，2017.

[21] Patricia M. Dillon. Nursing Health Assessment [M]. 2nd ed. Philadelphia: F. A. Davis, 2007.

[22] Paul L. Marino. The Little ICU Book of Facts and Formulas[M]. Philadelphia: Lippincott Williams & Wilkins, 2009.

[23] Linda Silvestri. Saunders Comprehensive Review for the NCLEX-RN® Examination [M]. London: Elsevier, 2019.

图书在版编目（CIP）数据

涉外护理情景模拟综合实训 = Nursing Simulations for Comprehensive Training : 英文 / 刘桂娟, 葛炜主编. — 杭州 : 浙江大学出版社, 2022.3

ISBN 978-7-308-22011-8

Ⅰ. ①涉… Ⅱ. ①刘… ②葛… Ⅲ. ①护理学－英语－口语－教材 Ⅳ. ①R47

中国版本图书馆CIP数据核字(2021)第243938号

涉外护理情景模拟综合实训

Nursing Simulations for Comprehensive Training

刘桂娟　葛　炜　主编

责任编辑　李　晨

责任校对　郑成业

封面设计　续设计

出版发行　浙江大学出版社

（杭州市天目山路148号　邮政编码　310007）

（网址：http：//www.zjupress.com）

排　　版　杭州林智广告有限公司

印　　刷　杭州宏雅印刷有限公司

开　　本　787mm×1092mm　1/16

印　　张　9

字　　数　200千

版 印 次　2022年3月第1版　2022年3月第1次印刷

书　　号　ISBN 978-7-308-22011-8

定　　价　30.00元
